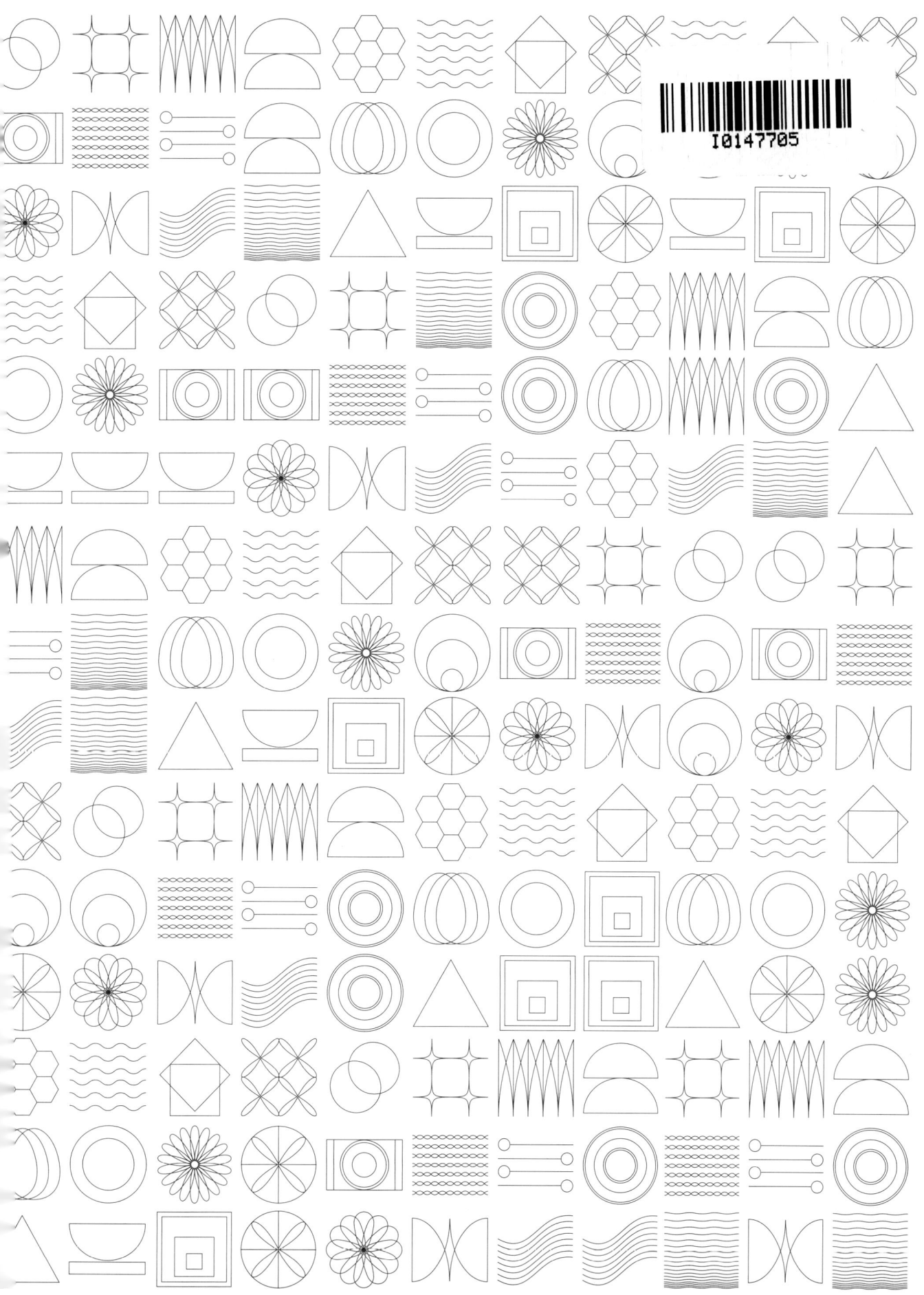

Women Who Heal

This book was written on the land of the Gadigal and Wangal people of the Eora Nation in Sydney, Australia. I pay respect to the past, present and future Traditional Custodians of these lands, waterways and skies.

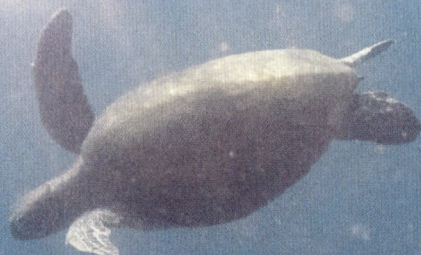

Women Who Heal

Natural practices for body and soul

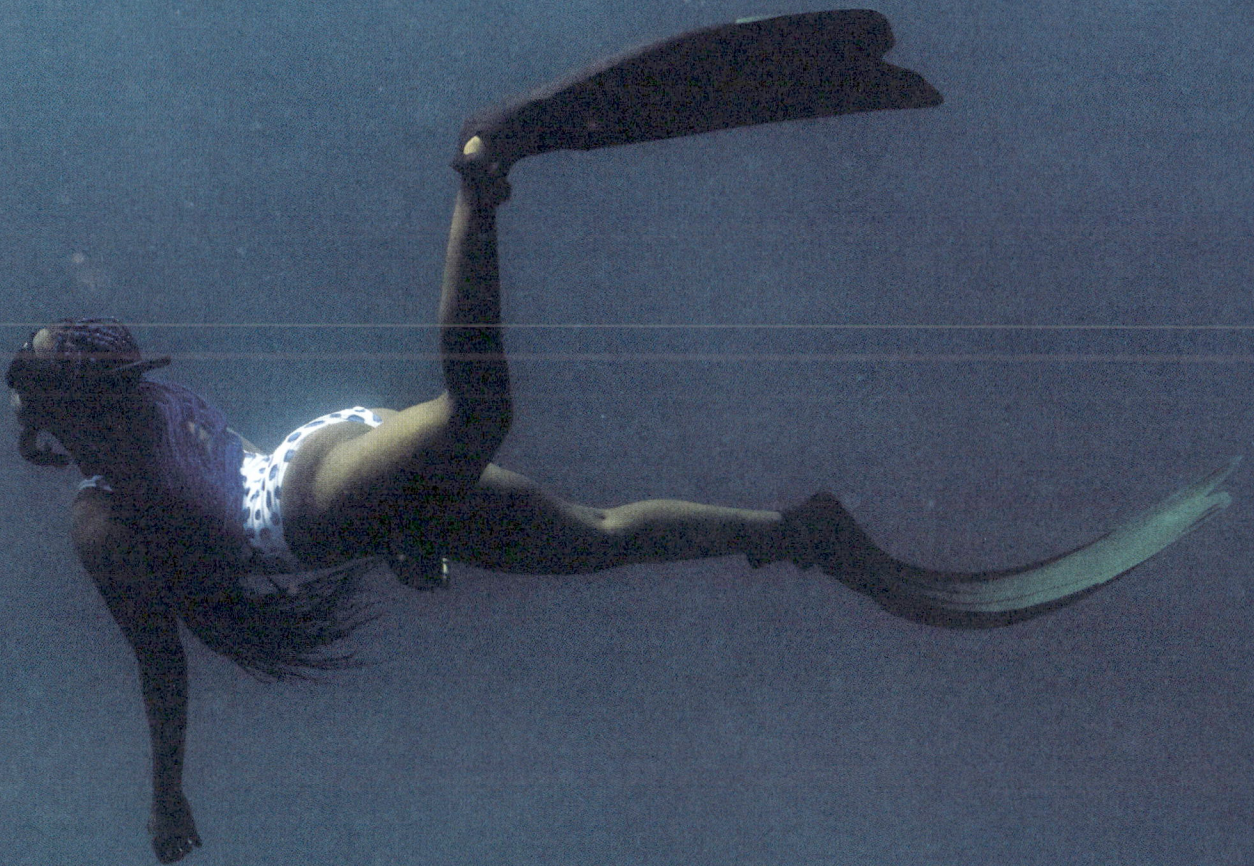

Emma Drady

B HLTHSC (NATUROPATHY)

T&H

Contents

Introduction 6

How you can use this book 9

The practice of nature 10

Cold-water exposure 12

Cold-water exposure for physical and mental health 20

Cooking 24

Farm to table 28

Wilderness immersion 34

Finding a sit spot to build a relationship with your local environment 38

Hiking 42

Surfing 46

Permaculture 52

Climate activism 58

The wisdom of nature 62

Herbalism 64

Plant meditation for feeling grounded and expansive 68

Beekeeping 72

Group adventures 78

Self-sufficient living 84

Veggie scrap broth for reducing waste 92

Farming 96

Textile design 102

Ocean education 106

Skin care 110

The wonder of nature 114

Flower growing 116

Art 120

• • • Nature drawing for exploring
your creativity 124

Mycology 128

Wildlife
photography 132

• • • Animal observation for
slowing down and cultivating
patience 136

Free diving 140

Art and design 146

Photography
and filmmaking 150

Floristry 156

Findings 162

Community 164

Curiosity 164

Healing 165

Patience 165

• • • Nature first-aid kit 166

For the now 168

For the future 170

Index of contributors 174

To the women 175

Acknowledgements 175

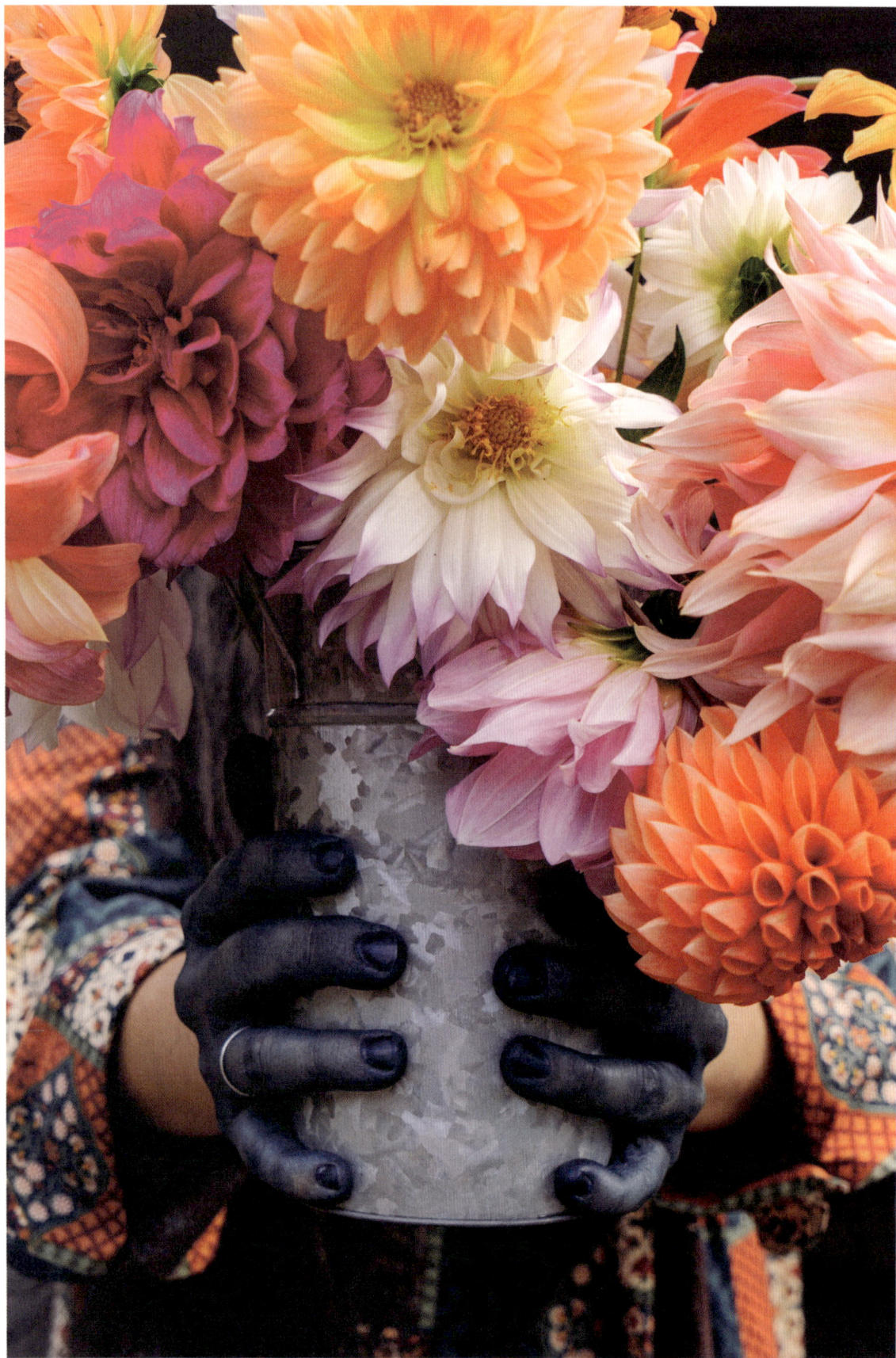

Introduction

Humans are a part of nature. But we have pushed it out, cut it down, tamed it, and disregarded its wisdom for such a long time that we now act as though we are entirely separate from it. It isn't until we have small moments, such as watching a particularly beautiful sunset or smelling that first scent of jasmine at the start of spring, that we recognise how wired we are to appreciate the beauty of the natural world.

Finding the time to sit outdoors or take long meandering hikes through the bush can be challenging when trying to keep up with the expectations of work and personal life. It can be easy to fall into the cyclical and often monotonous sleep-eat-work-repeat routine. When you have been inside for too long – perhaps it has been raining for days or your work schedule is demanding – that first re-emergence out into the sun and the fresh air can feel completely invigorating.

My job as a naturopath is to support people, predominantly women, with their health. I use the term 'woman' to refer to those who are both assigned female at birth and those who identify as women. These patients may have digestive complaints, sleep struggles, irregular menstrual cycles, weakened immune systems and other physical ailments that they are seeking respite from. I wholeheartedly want to help these people with their physical health, but the more I practise and the longer that I am doing this job, I have come to realise that there are so many other facets that come into play: our mental and emotional health; our relationships; our ability to express ourselves creatively; our sense of community and purpose; and then what I deem to be the missing piece of the puzzle, our connection with nature.

When someone is sitting across from me in the clinic, I am often their last resort. They have likely tried all kinds of things with little to no improvements. Many of these patients have hit a standstill in their progress or have been putting up with mediocre health for too long. In these circumstances I find myself more frequently prescribing 'getting out into nature'. I've told patients to take off their shoes more often outside, I've suggested a walk around the block in the sunshine

$\longrightarrow$

on lunch breaks, I've even told someone they have to go on a bushwalk before their next appointment just to get them out the door. For the ones willing to pursue these paths, the transformation occurs. Nature is, time and time again, the missing link.

In life (and naturopathy) there is no one size fits all, so I began exploring what other women were doing to connect more deeply with nature. Where did their relationship to plants, animals or water begin? How did they feel when they first started? What benefits have they noticed? My inquisitive nature took me to artists, survival skills experts, chefs, farmers and many others who have helped me build up my naturopathic dispensary of nature prescriptions. And so, here are the stories of twenty-five inspiring relationships with the natural world. My hopes are that someone in these pages and the prescriptions I have written will ignite a desire to try something new or reconnect with an old practice.

Nature is about balance. There is no 'all or nothing' in nature, there is harmony. This is also how we should approach health. We don't need to move to the forest and away from our jobs and families to have a connection with nature. Just as we don't need to completely banish lazy days or pizza nights to be healthy. You are a part of nature. By connecting more with nature, you will connect with yourself.

Keep this book in close reach so that when you feel that spark within you to connect more with nature, you can return to these pages knowing you now have the tools.

How you can use this book

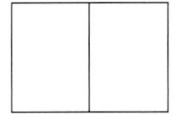

1. The stories and sections

This book is an opportunity to learn from and be inspired by women who have walked unmarked paths and persevered in pursuits totally outside of their comfort zones. When we see an example of someone doing something we had never dreamed of, it gives us hope and perhaps a little 'well if she can do it, so can I' gusto.

The book is divided into three sections: the practice of nature, the wisdom of nature and the wonder of nature. The practice of nature includes women who are using nature in a practical way. These stories would be helpful for people who are more logical and action oriented. The wisdom of nature includes stories from women who have learnt something from nature and would appeal to people who like to understand and take deeper meaning from their experiences. The wonder of nature features women who have been inspired by nature and are typically a more creative cohort. This is for people who like a more spiritual or beauty-driven theme.

You may be drawn to a particular story or section, but I implore you to read widely – you never know what might resonate with you.

2. Prescriptions

Woven throughout the stories and inspired by the women, are six prescriptions or activities to try. I have given an explanation as to why this activity may be useful, as well as a step-by-step guide for how you can try it at home.

These activities are all safe and easy to do. In fact, I regularly prescribe activities just like these in my naturopathy practice as part of a holistic treatment plan. I recommend trying each of them as you go along. Return to your favourites and work towards incorporating them into your everyday life. Before you know it, you will be immersed in nature daily without even trying.

3. Nature first-aid kit

At the back of this book I have created a list of nature-based remedies to help a variety of ailments (see page 167). Whether you are a single mum working full-time with a lot on your plate, a teenager exploring a connection to nature for the first time, or any woman in between or outside of these scopes, there is something here for you.

I have broken down these remedies into 'for the now' and 'for the future'. If you are currently experiencing symptoms and are looking to alleviate some of your discomfort, the 'for the now' section will have some options for instant relief. For prevention, I suggest exploring and implementing the items from 'for the future'.

The practice of nature

The relationship between nature and humans is long ingrained. Before we had infrastructure and technology, we lived immersed in the natural world. Our shelter, our sustenance and our livelihoods all depended on learning techniques to survive in nature.

We learnt how to harvest from nature – to tame it so that it benefited us. The practices we developed were part survival and part progress, for ourselves and the natural environment. We understood that without nature, we wouldn't survive.

Our ancestors had a deep respect for nature. Many traditional practices acknowledge that rather than taking everything we can see, we must also leave some behind. Reciprocity is a practice that allows us to benefit from nature by not only helping it to regenerate but to flourish.

In our modern world, we now have survival covered and so we have the opportunity to turn our attention to nature for recreation and pleasure. Practices that may have been a waste of energy for our earliest humans are now a source of our wellbeing and part of our daily lives.

Human evolution has seen our basic needs expand beyond food, water and shelter. Psychologists and social scientists now recognise that we also need a sense of purpose, significance and variety in our life to feel fulfilled: climbing a mountain, riding a wave, eating for flavour. To practise is to do something repeatedly. And to repeatedly return to and care for nature can be a practice in itself.

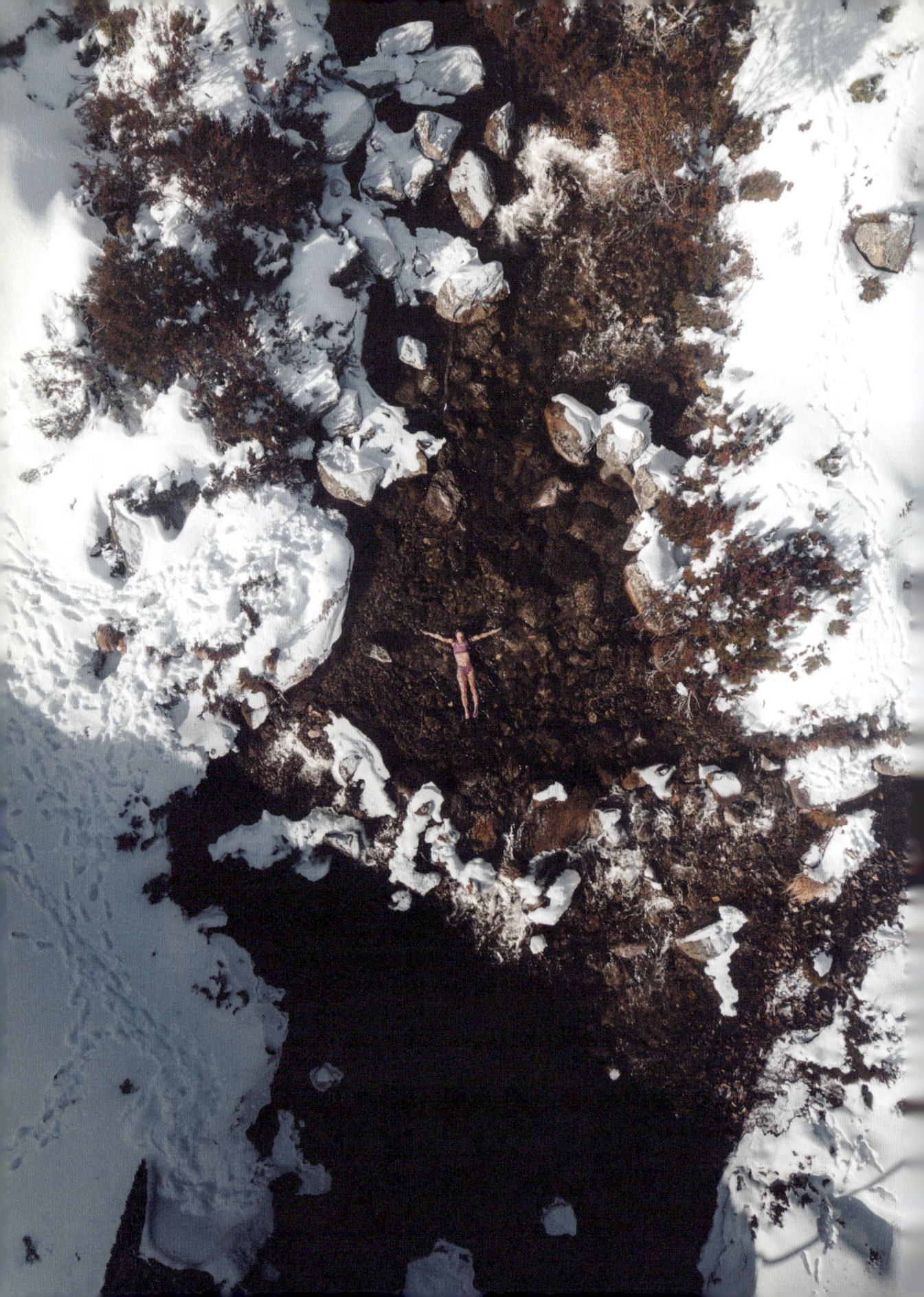

Cold-water exposure

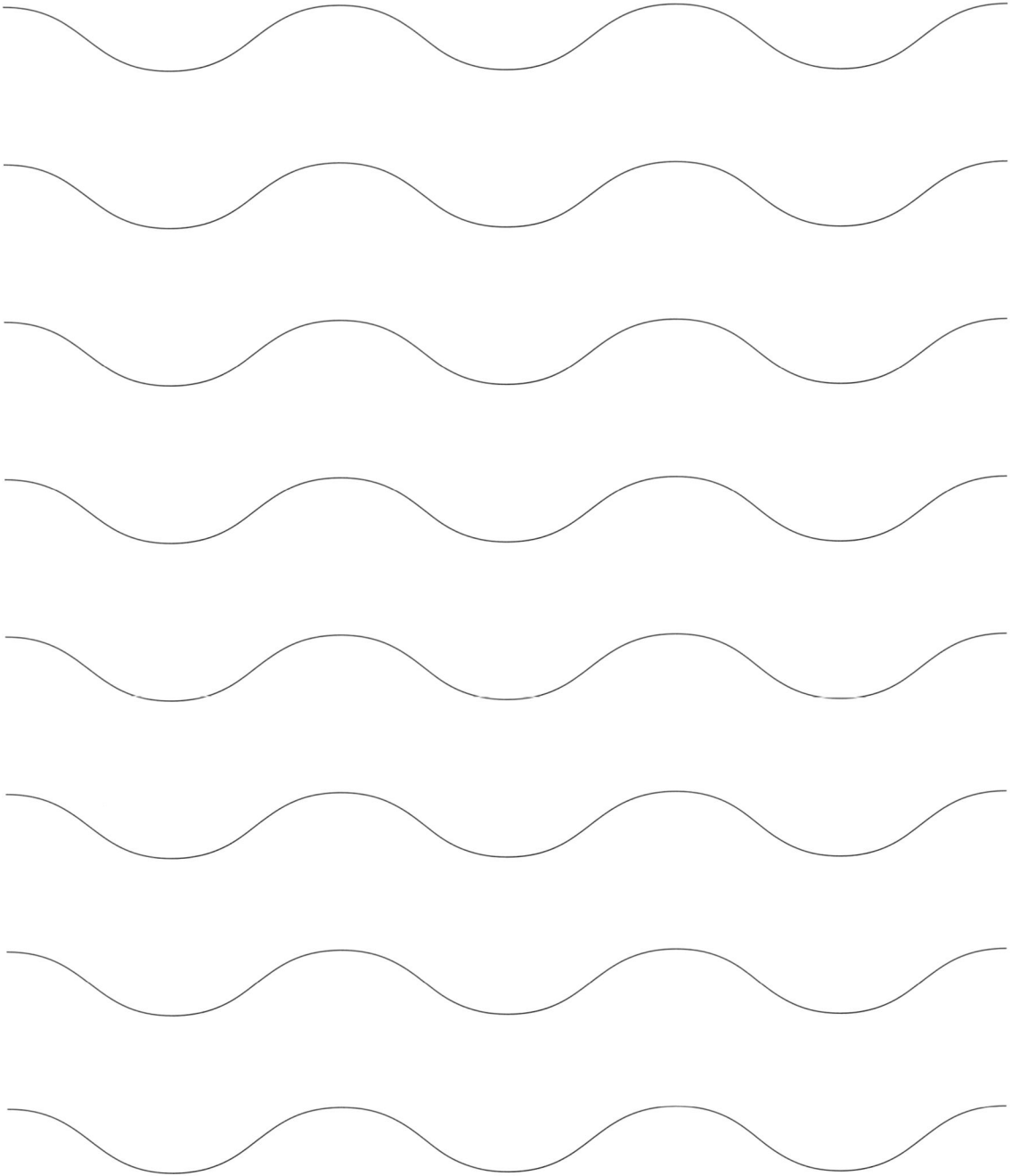

Using cold-water therapy to enhance overall health

Leah Scott

● Australia

Following the divorce from her husband, Leah fell into a spiral of extreme anxiety, stress and depression. At her self-described rock bottom, Leah realised she needed to make a change and began exploring different healing modalities.

This search led her to the Wim Hof Method, a combination of breathing techniques and cold-water exposure. Describing her first experience as euphoric and beautiful, Leah came out of it feeling at peace for the first time in over a year. She was hooked, and within two months Leah experienced a strong pull to explore her limits with the cold, prompting her to move to one of the coldest parts of the country.

Leah grew up in Queensland, Australia, and remembers as a young child being whisked off to waterfalls and rivers on the weekends by her parents. She always felt a strong connection to nature but, like many of us, her priorities shifted when she grew older and became more social as a teenager and then later as a wife and mother. 'Culture and society wanted me to have those priorities,' she says. 'Everything was structured, but I realised that once I started ticking off all of the goals, there was no pot of gold at the end.'

From her new balcony, Leah could see Lake Jindabyne and she began to go down there regularly. 'I would drive down every morning, sometimes it would be snowing, and I would strip off and go into the river,' says Leah. During one of these early experiences, Leah had what she describes as a spiritual encounter. She felt a separateness from her thoughts, her body and her mind, and became one with the river. Describing it as a gift, she realised she needed to share this experience with others. 'It's changed every single perception in my life, even the way I raise my children. I'm calm, I'm patient, I'm peaceful.'

The transformations that Leah has witnessed, both personally and in the retreats she leads, are profound. 'To see how we react in a difficult environment really highlights how we live in the world,' says Leah. Fear of the cold is passed on very early. As children we are told to put a jumper on and stay warm, but releasing that fear and going into the water surrounded by ice is how Leah helps her retreat attendees create distance from their thoughts and let go of their trepidations.

'Yes, it can hurt. The body is sweating and the pupils are dilated, but after about sixty to ninety seconds there is a wave of calmness in the chaos as stress is released from the body.' Coming out of the icy water then gives the body a dopamine hit (the hormone released to signal pleasure) – a reward for conquering your fear and moving through limiting beliefs, which can be life changing.

Leah facilitates retreats for all people but her all-female groups are her favourites. She notices that while some are very happy to just jump straight into the water, others often take their time in understanding the weight of the experience as more than just a physical challenge. Slowing down becomes part of the experience. 'The world is fast, but nature is not in a rush, she's so slow. She's the opposite of the structured social world,' says Leah. 'We women should be in flow. Attuning to nature at a deeper level and spending time within it teaches us to let go.'

The practice of nature

Revisiting the memory of sitting by a river on an early morning where everything was white and still among the snow, Leah recalls being visited by a rust-coloured fox that came down for a drink and stopped just metres from her across the bank. For a minute or two the fox just stood there looking Leah in the eyes before walking back into the snow. Moments like this are what made all her sacrifices over the years worth it for her. 'For a while it was an incredibly lonely journey, but I had the deepest knowing that I had to do this,' says Leah referring to a time before her retreats. 'I received a message of how many lives I could help change if I just kept going. It felt like a sacrifice then but there was never any going back.'

Leah now finds great peace hiking mountains and sleeping under the stars. She describes one of her greatest lessons from nature as the feeling of freedom. 'Nature has allowed me to slow down because when I'm out there I become nature.'

'When we go out into nature, we can observe our true selves.'

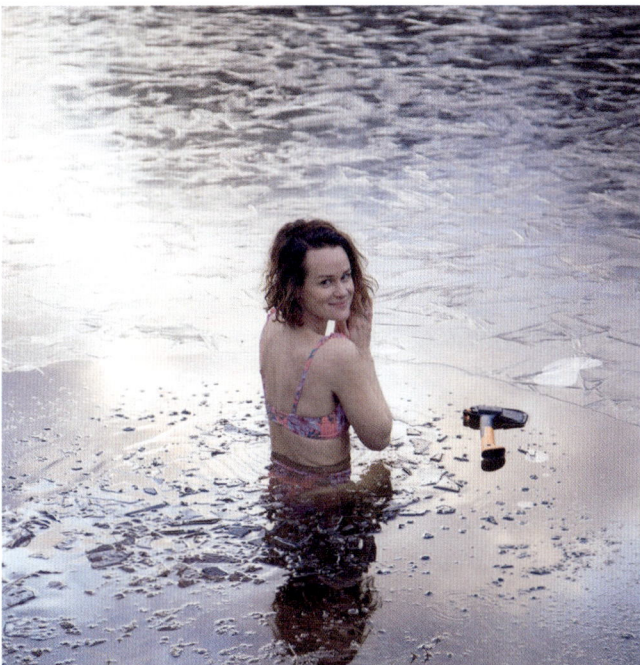

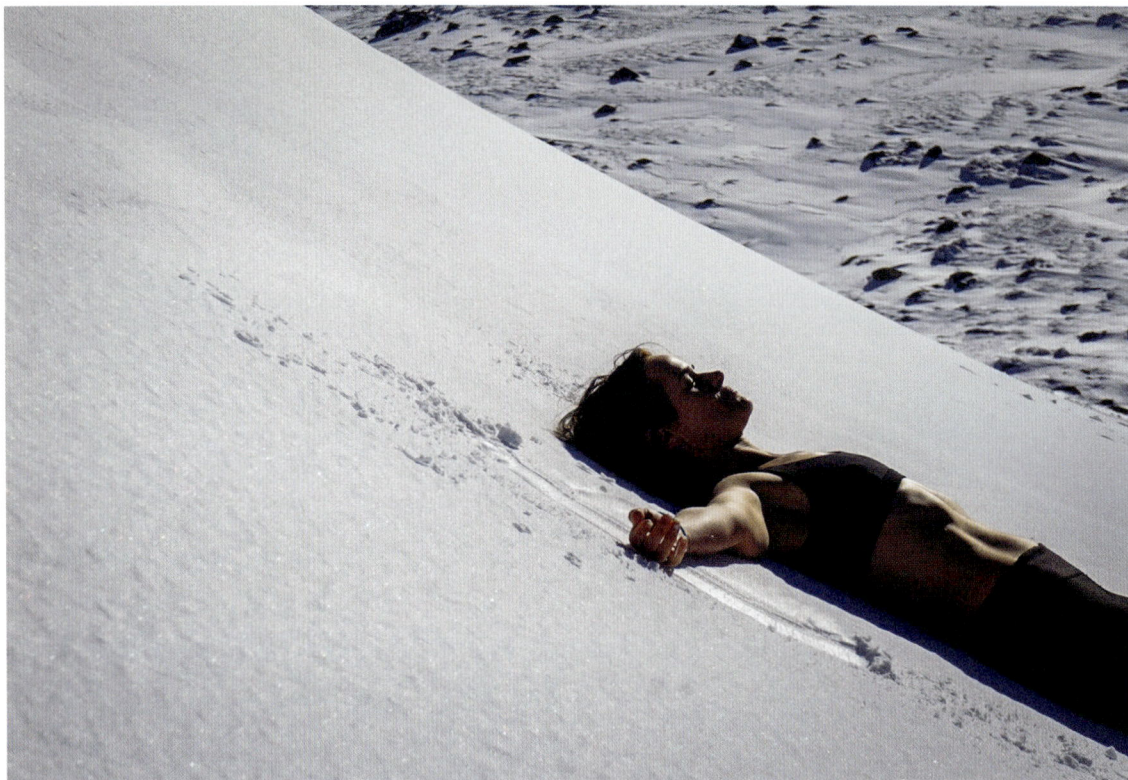

≋ 'The world is fast, but nature is not in a rush, she's so slow.
She's the opposite of the structured social world.'
– Leah Scott

The practice of nature

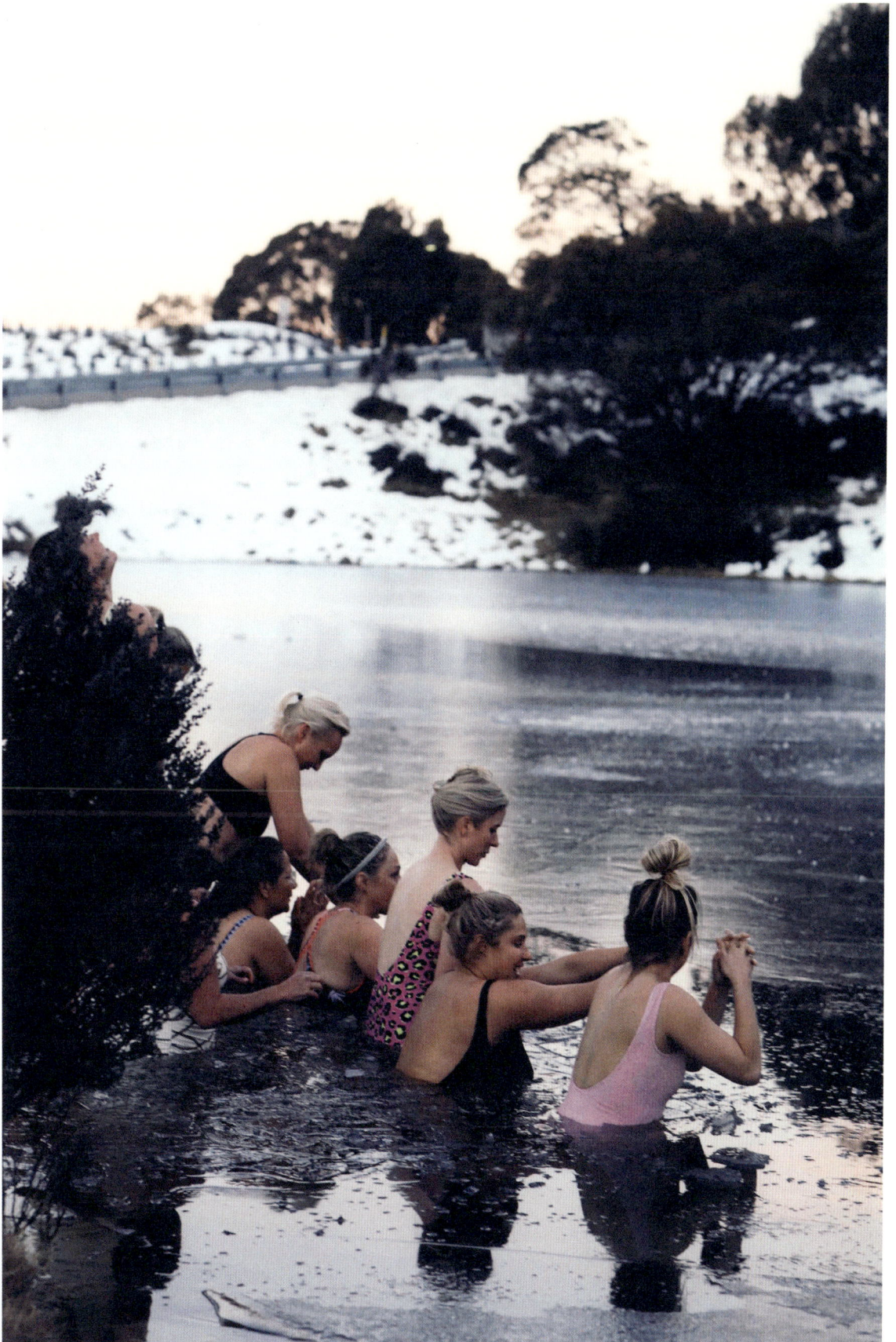

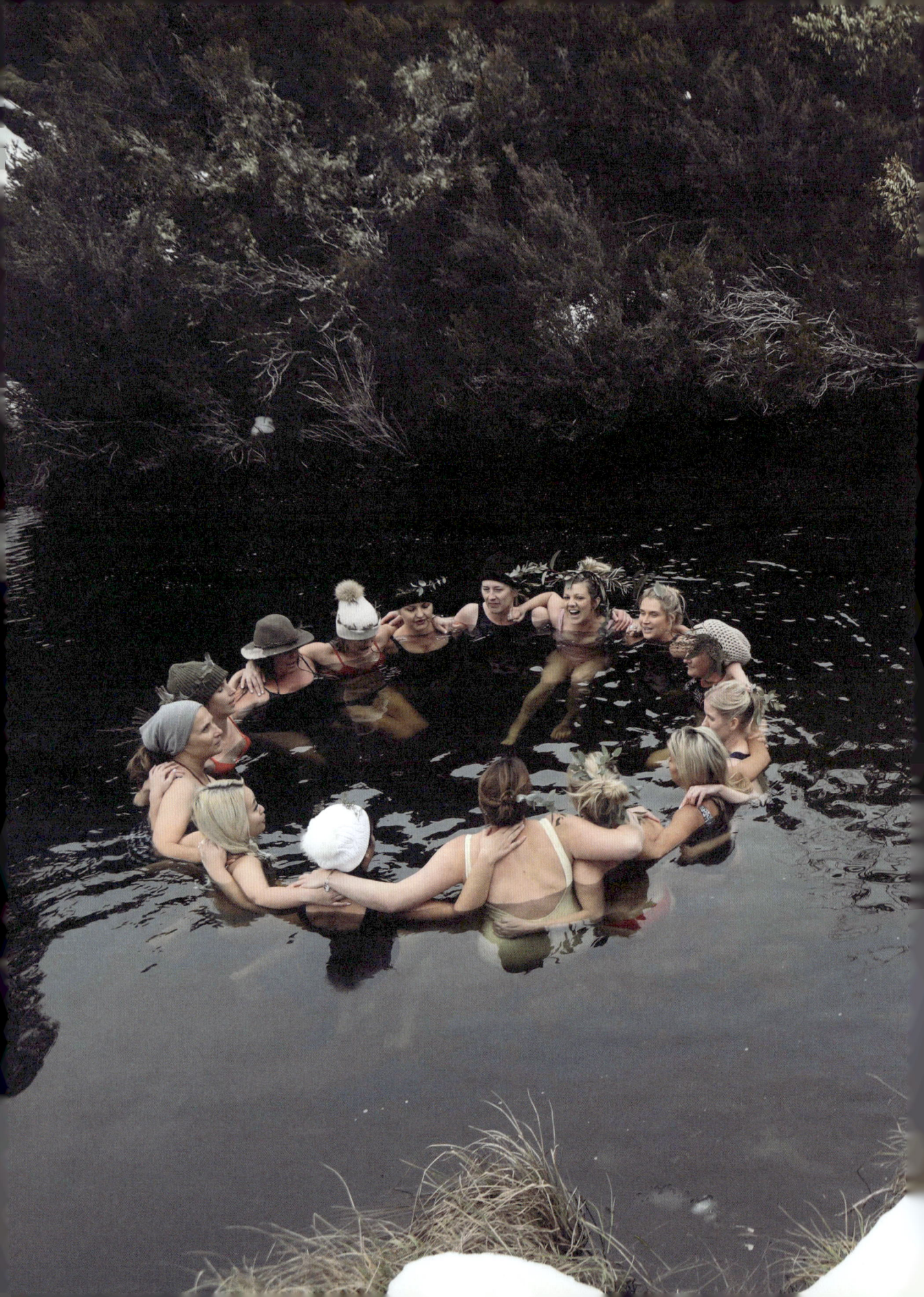

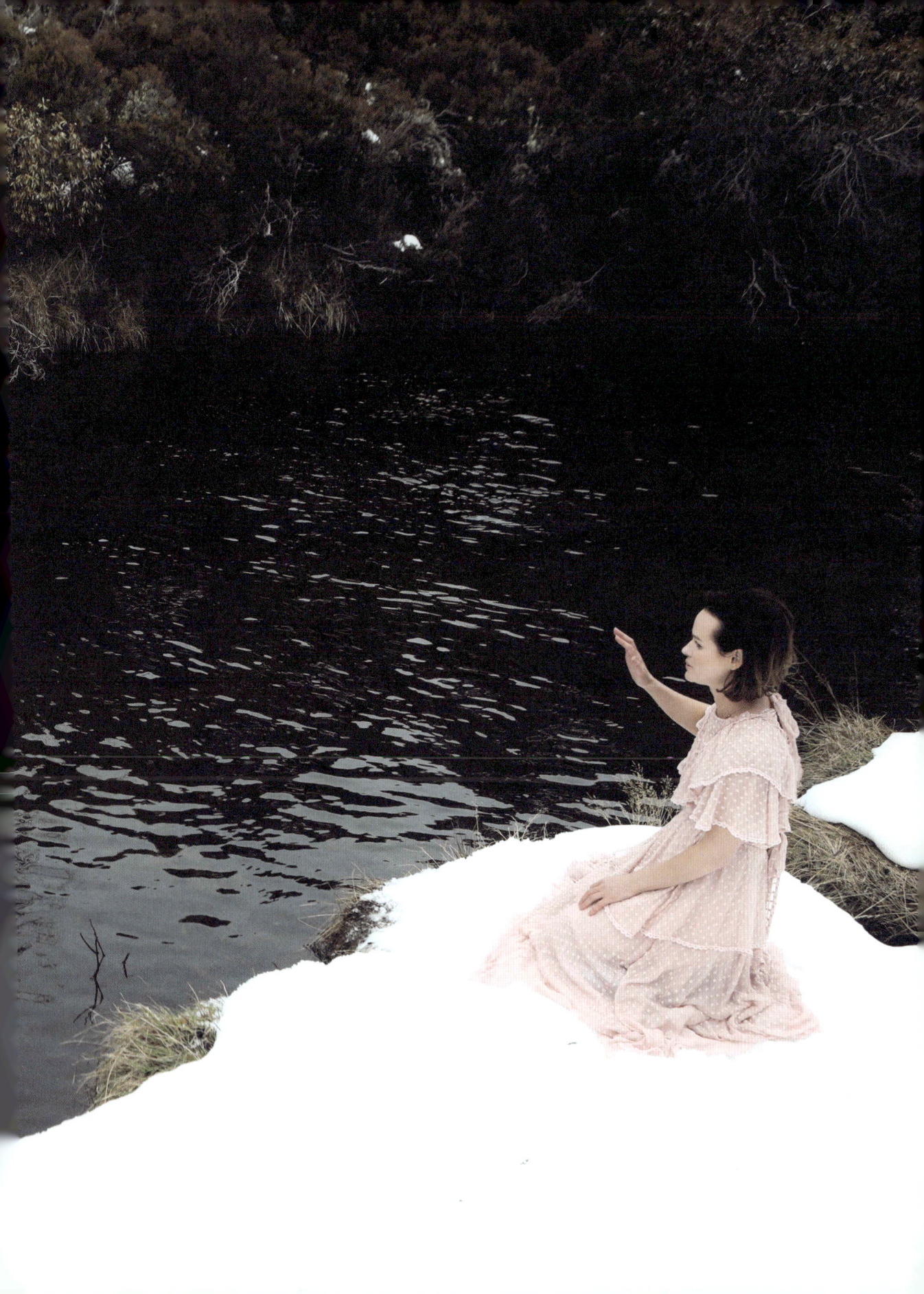

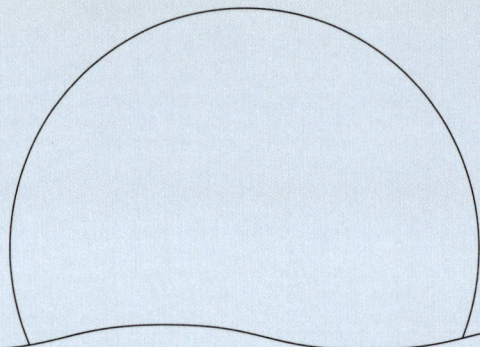

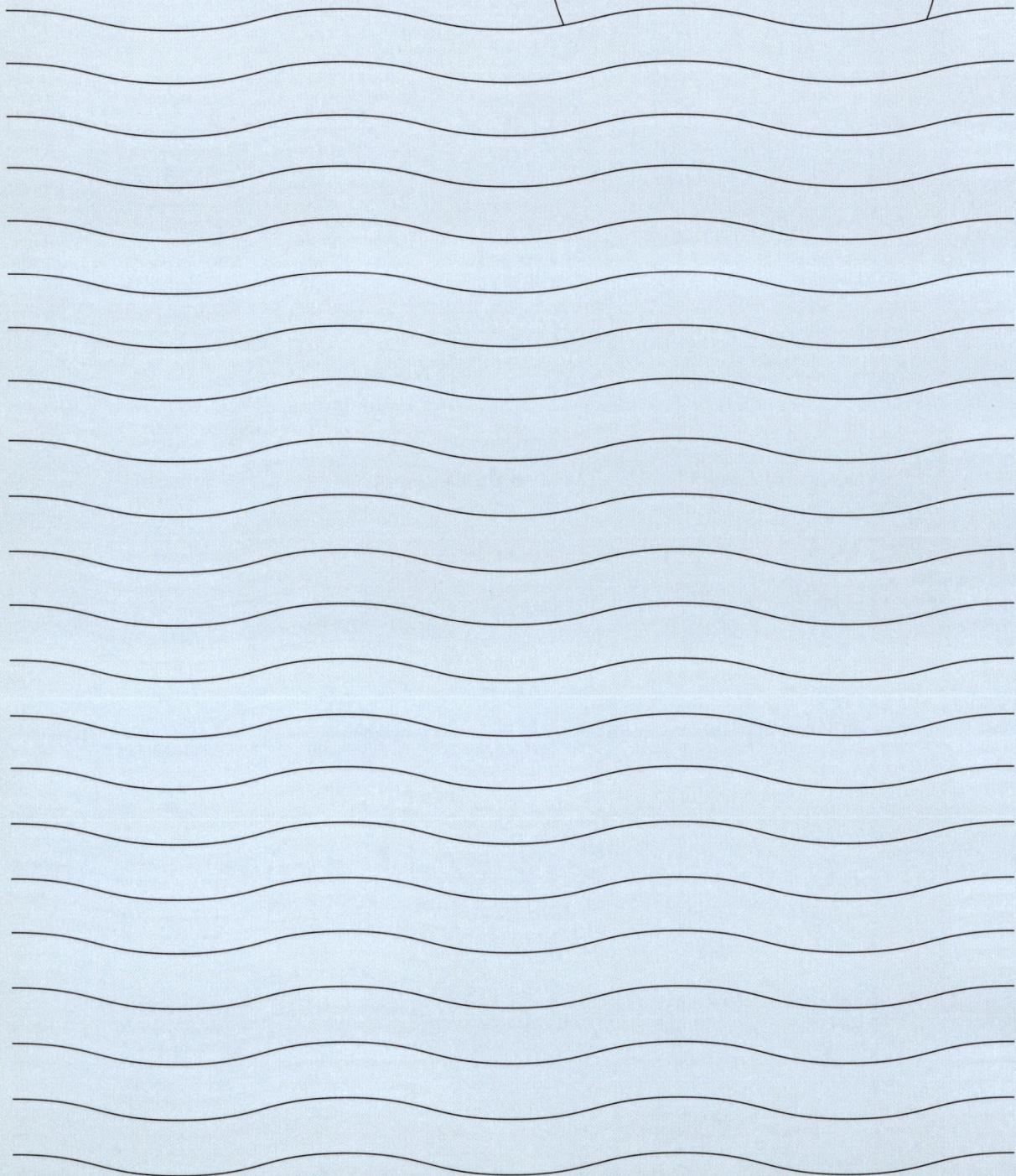

Cold-water exposure for physical and mental health

Inspired by Leah Scott

Cold-water swimming has been practised throughout Scandinavia, the Baltics and Russia since at least the 18th century. Popularised in the last decade, in large part due to the work of Wim Hof, the Dutch 'ice man', who has been guiding people all over the world into icy plunges and snow walks. Many of the understood health benefits are thanks to Hof's willingness to be studied and the upholding of traditions from these northern countries.

Science has slowly been catching up with these practices, showing us that immersing our bodies in cold water can:

- improve blood pressure and circulation
- quicken muscle recovery in athletes
- strengthen the immune system
- support the body's metabolism
- have profound impacts on mental health – there have now been multiple reports of patients with treatment-resistant depression making full recoveries and even leading to a discontinuation of medication for some.

It sounds almost too good to be true. Could a simple dunk in the pool or a bath filled with icy water really be a solution to so many of our major health concerns? There isn't anything more potent for refreshing the body and mind than the feeling of diving underwater. No need to worry if natural open water is not something you have access to as bathtubs, showers and even splashing your face with cold water have also been shown to provide positive benefits.

$\longrightarrow$

To begin ●

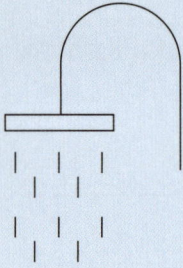

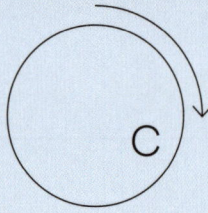

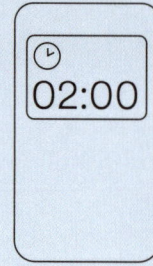

●1
Start by gradually introducing colder water at the end of your shower.

●2
Each time you reduce the temperature, allow yourself a few moments to adjust before lowering the temperature further.

●3
If you are struggling to adjust to the cold, you are at the temperature where the most health benefits are found.
Try to stay with it for a minute or two.

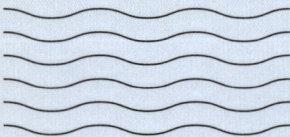

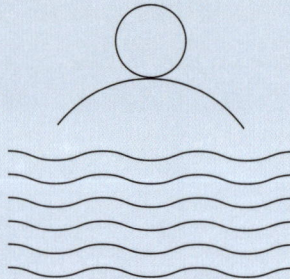

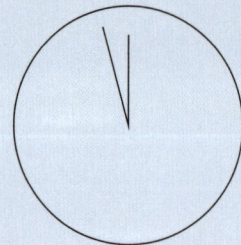

●7
Firstly, you want to try to calm your nervous system by taking some deep breaths, concentrating on elongating your exhale.

●8
When you are feeling calmer, enter the water on the exhale. Don't put your head under if the water is freezing over. Always have someone with you if there is snow, ice or this is the first time you are doing it.

●9
The first minute is always the hardest, breathe through it.

The practice of nature

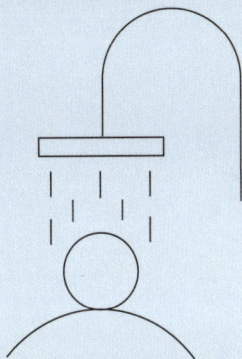

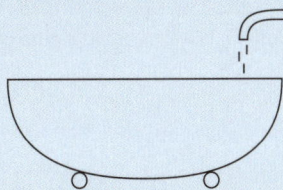

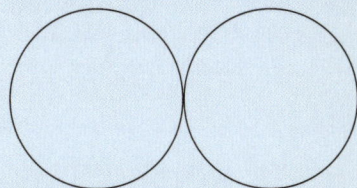

4

Eventually you will be able to begin your showers from a colder temperature or go completely cold the whole time.

5

You might find that this is enough for you, which is great. Otherwise, once you have been doing this practice for a while and feel you are ready to try the next stage, decide where you would like to do your plunge. A bath or large tub of cold water works just as well as a lake, river or ocean.

6

Find someone to be there with you who will stay out of the water for words of encouragement and support should you need it.

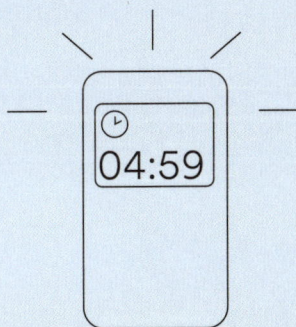

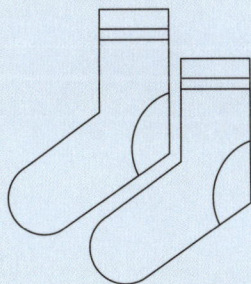

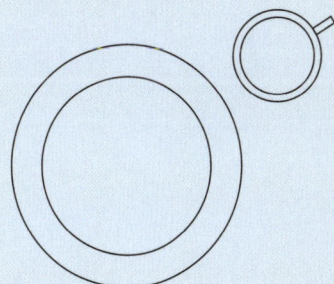

10

Five minutes is your sweet spot. If you can stay in the water for this long, your body will be getting the most benefits. If you are really struggling, get out and try again another time.

11

Be sure to warm up as soon as you get out of the water with dry clothes, socks, gloves and a hat.

12

Drink warm tea and have something to eat. Don't have a hot shower as the sudden change in temperature can be a shock to the system.

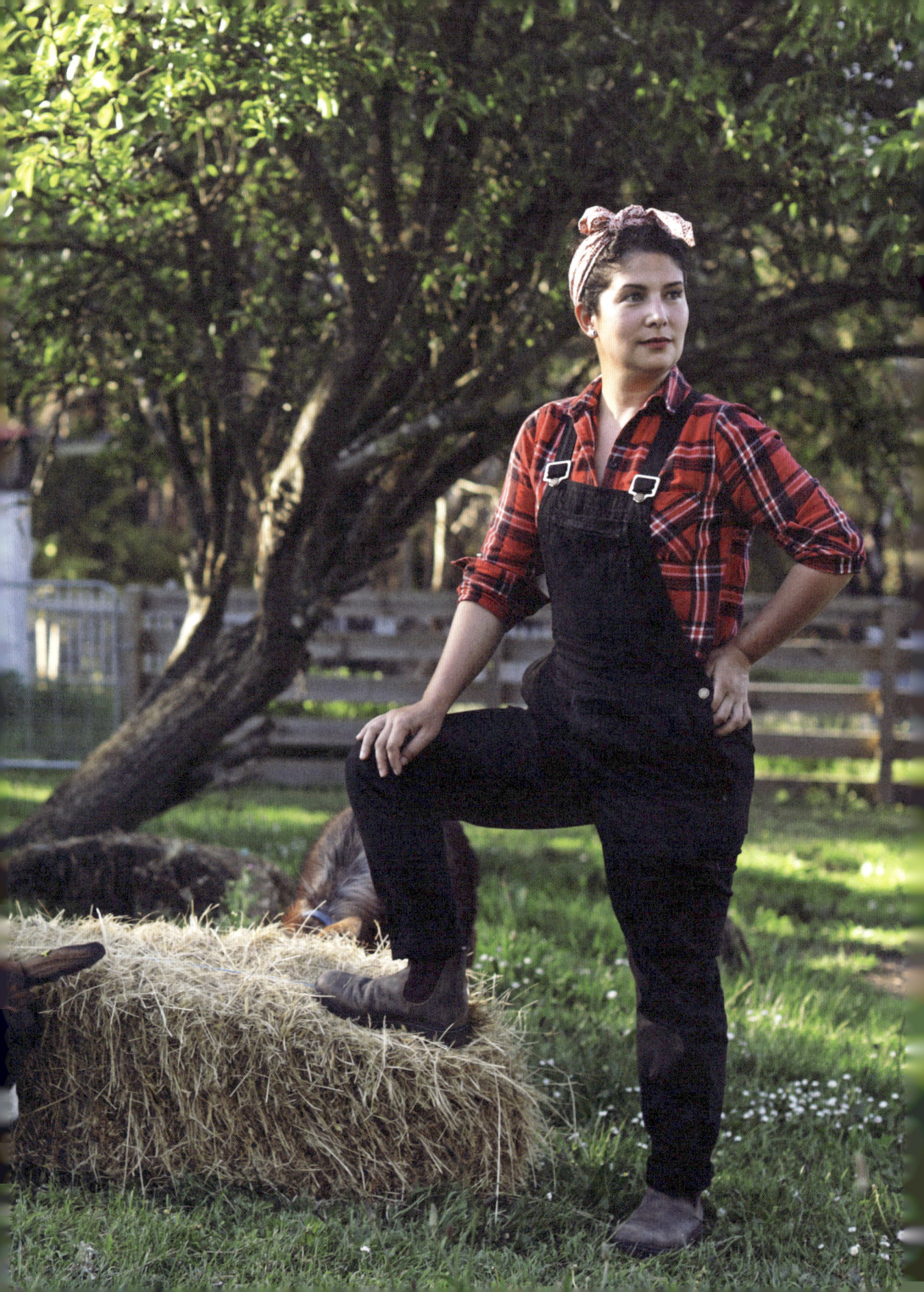

Cooking

Using local ingredients to foster appreciation

Analiese Gregory

● Australia

Long hours and stress are part of the reason why Analiese made a radical change to her life. She had been on a steady career path as a chef but, after working very intense sixteen-to-eighteen hour days, she had the thought of leaving and living in the French countryside and in 2012 she did just that. She landed at Bras restaurant in southern France, famed for its homegrown and forage-inspired menu, including their version of *gargouillou* – a salad featuring over sixty different flowers, herbs and vegetables.

While at the restaurant, Analiese spent the mornings picking produce from the chef's garden and going foraging in the afternoons. 'I spent all my time hiking trails, looking for rare flowers, wood sorrel and things like that. I'd put headphones on and take a baguette, cheese and sometimes wine with me. I spent a really beautiful year just immersed in that.'

Having had a taste of a different pace of life, Analiese found herself seeking out more experiences where she could spend time outdoors. This is how she eventually ended up landing at the very bottom of the world in Tasmania, Australia. Originally intending to stay for six months, five years later she is still there. Stepping away from the order and rigidity of Michelin-starred restaurants, she is now picking wild wakame (seaweed), hunting wallabies and foraging mushrooms. This has been a welcome change not only to how she cooks but how she lives her life.

'There used to be a lot of convenience in my life because I worked so much, but now, with this lifestyle, you have to physically do everything yourself. If I want the house to be warm, I have to light a wood fire, so I need to have wood ... and in different sizes ... and it needs to be dry. My life is entirely different now.'

Analiese is much more intentional with the way she selects her produce, choosing local as much as possible and building relationships with the growers. This is partly because of the freshness but also due to her new-found understanding of the challenges involved in farming. 'It's a difficult subject for me. I had a veggie garden, but it got decimated by rabbits and possums two or three times. So now it's very well fenced and netted, and I'm slowly starting again. It's been a lesson: don't go too big too soon.'

With this new knowledge of growing, it's hard to believe the waste she witnessed in so many of the high-end restaurants she previously worked in. 'A place I worked at in Paris would order twenty bunches of asparagus. We'd then pick out ten bunches that were all the same size and send the others back just to get them all identical,' she says. A far cry from the excitement she now feels seeing the season's first asparagus spears bursting through the soil in the garden.

Analiese remembers spending time with her Cantonese grandmother as a child and learning how to make pork buns and mapo tofu as well as picking flowers in her childhood garden. But that was the extent of her cooking and experiences in nature growing up. She highlights that her current way of life has been a very conscious decision that she's made in her adulthood. 'If I can do this coming from

The practice of nature

living in big cities, not owning a car and a life of 24-hour supermarkets and restaurants, anyone can. You can make a decision about what you want in your life and just pursue it.'

The adjustment has not always been easy, but over time Analiese has felt her body slowly adapting to the cycles of nature. 'Living in the countryside, it's dark at night-time and nothing happens. I now know why people go to bed and get up early – you can get more done. I had never thought of that when I was working until 11 pm or midnight in fluorescent lighting.' After a year, everything began to reset and although she is still busy – renovating her home and shed into a ten-seater restaurant, filming a television show and writing a second book – it is in a different way. She has felt her health improve and many of her initial worries of being isolated and alone are subsiding as she immerses herself in the local community.

Having gone on this journey and felt the benefits, Analiese wants people to think of the last time they remember enjoying themselves. 'Think about your responses and if a lot of the answers are based outdoors, then that's probably a path you should go down. Work to have more of that in your life.'

'If you can do something that makes you feel better about yourself and the world, and you can collect food at the same time, it feels like a win-win situation.'

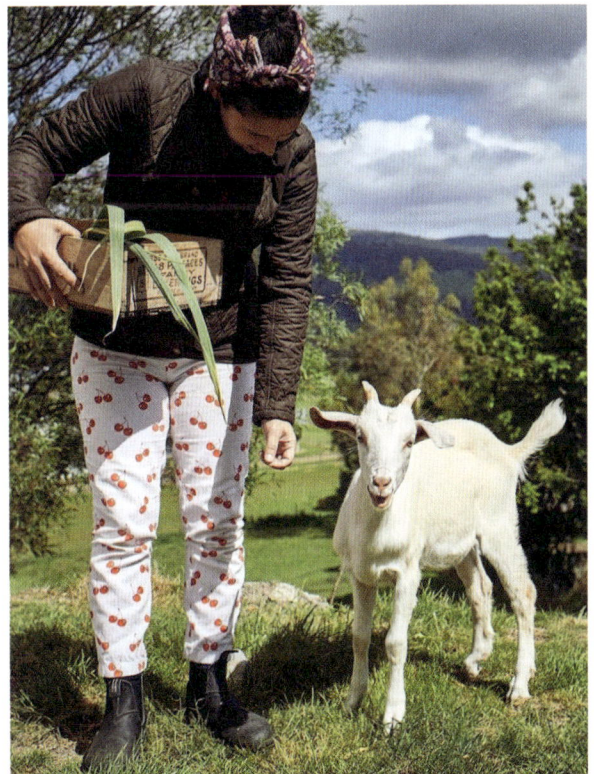

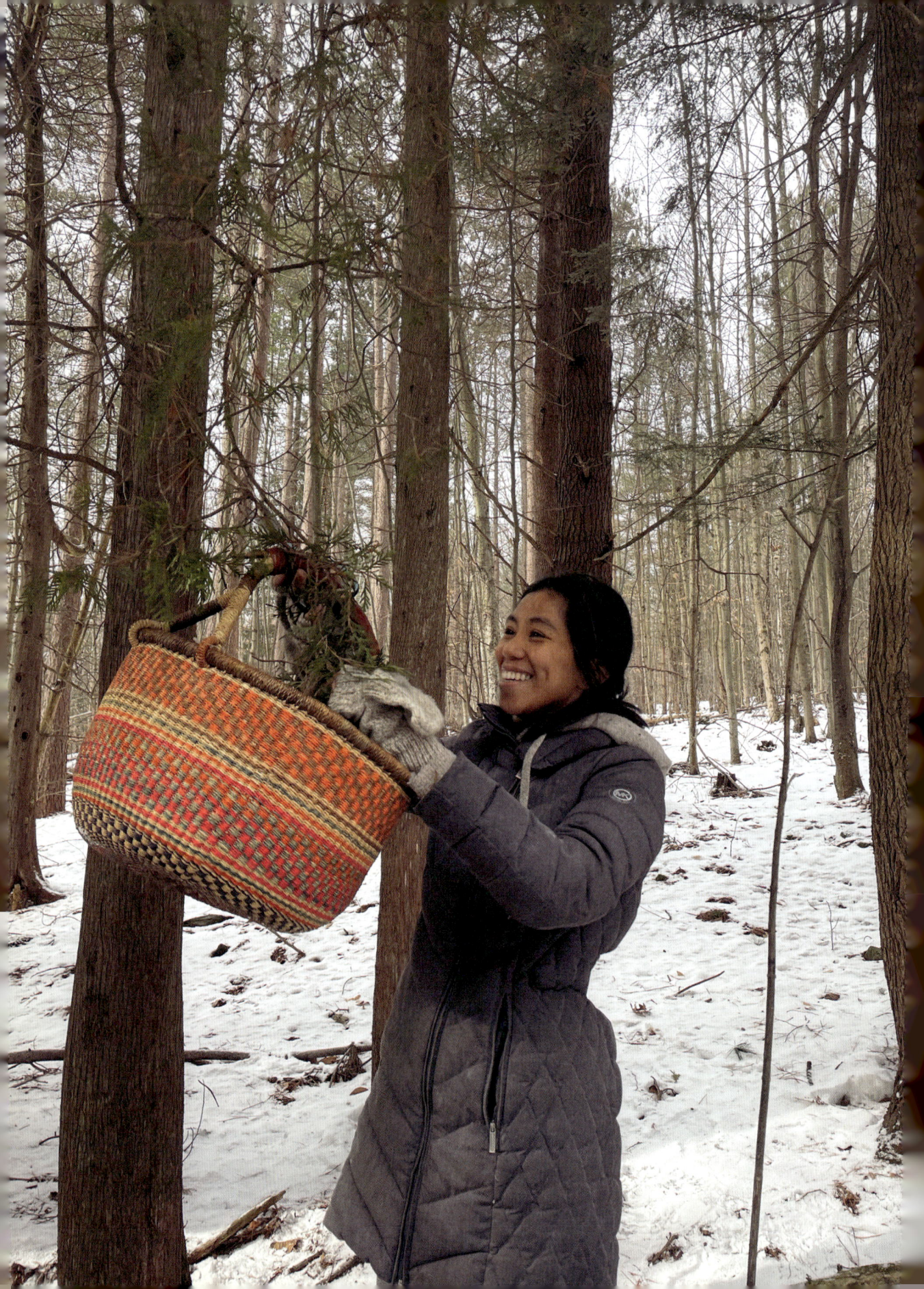

Farm to table

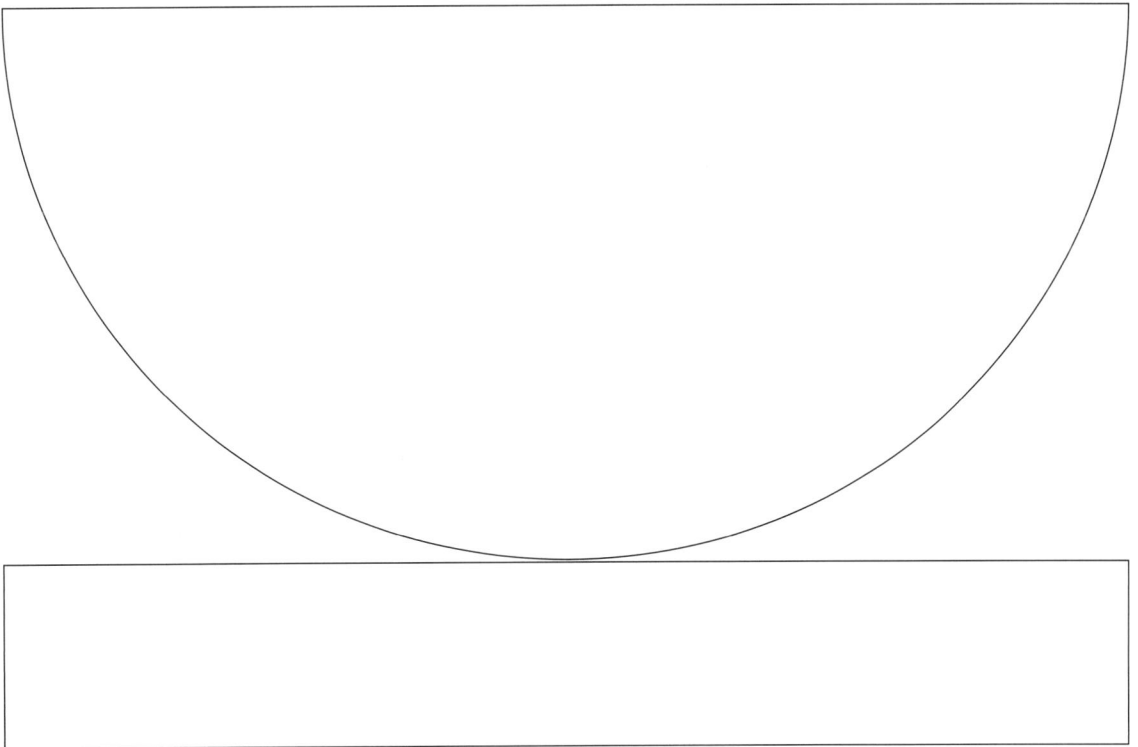

Understanding the seasons to reduce food waste

Ria Ibrahim Taylor

● USA

As the farm-to-table manager at Soul Fire Farm, Ria Ibrahim Taylor works in a yearly cycle of planting, harvesting, collecting seeds and preserving in order to reduce not only food wastage but shortages during the winter months. Although, it has been a big adjustment from the heat and sun she was familiar with in Indonesia, moving to upstate New York, USA, and living with four seasons has been one of the most profound lessons for her.

Farm to table is about finding local food for cooking as close as possible to the source. It aims to provide the freshest possible ingredients as well as reduce the environmental impact of transportation and wastage. As an example of this, Ria explains that in summer they grow delicious red tomatoes, but in autumn the remaining tomatoes are still green. In an effort to reduce food waste, they made approximately 23 kilograms of green tomato sambal last season.

Along with cooking for the staff and guests at Soul Fire's workshops and weekend immersions, Ria helps to determine what will be grown the following season. 'The farm manager and I will work out what crops did and didn't go well because of the weather and soil. We work together to decide so I can create the menu,' she says. Ria's aim is that 85 per cent of the ingredients they use in their meals are from the farm.

Initially this was a challenge for Ria who loves to cook Asian-inspired food from her home country of Indonesia. Many of her favourite spices, like lemongrass and ginger, don't always grow well with the shorter seasons in her new climate. 'I didn't want to always buy things from an Asian supermarket and for ingredients to travel far across the country. So we grow things from seed and put it in a high tunnel (a microclimate structure like a greenhouse).' This allows Ria to grow some of her favourite plants that would otherwise not survive.

Coming from a family of black pepper and vanilla farmers, Ria learnt how to harvest and prepare food from a young age. 'In South Sulawesi, where I grew up, everyone had to grow and cook their own food,' she says. 'The ground there was like red clay. My friend and I would make pots from it and pretend we were cooking, just like our mums.' Eventually Ria's mum and grandma taught her about different herbs and why it was so important to know how to grow food for yourself. 'Growing up, my mum always said that if you know how to grow and cook your own food, you can be very independent in society and also help others.'

Ria is now passing on some of this knowledge to her daughter who comes farming and foraging with her. 'She's really good at identifying turkey tail mushrooms. She knows how to harvest tomatoes and how to identify wild berries that can be eaten.' At just four years old, Ria's daughter is already showing signs of her understanding of where food really comes from. 'When we go to the grocery store, she asks, "Why are the eggs in there Mummy, where are the chickens?"' A simple question, but one that many children in urban and suburban environments may never have asked.

This is one of the reasons why Soul Fire Farm has started their program 'Soul Fire in the City'. An initiative to help people in cities connect to the food cycle and learn how to grow their own crops. 'A program team will go to vacant lots in the city. We build raised beds and bring seedlings or seeds and train them how to grow their food,' says Ria. Having food sovereignty is one of the main aims of Soul Fire Farm, particularly for people of colour and youth. Their mission is to provide education and access to growing food to all people, no matter your gender, race or background.

In her spare time Ria likes to while away the hours in nature by foraging and walking. 'When I'm in the forest I'm very tuned in. It's easy to see the wind and the light between the branches. It's like a Mary Oliver poem when I'm among the trees,' she says. The similarities between Earth and motherhood is something that Ria has witnessed since having her daughter. She continues to pull from this in her farm-to-table work. 'When I see my daughter all I want is to love her. And when I'm working with nature, I also want to provide the best. To protect Mother Nature. It's the same as how I want to be with my daughter.'

'If you know how to grow and cook your own food, you can be very independent in society and also help others.'

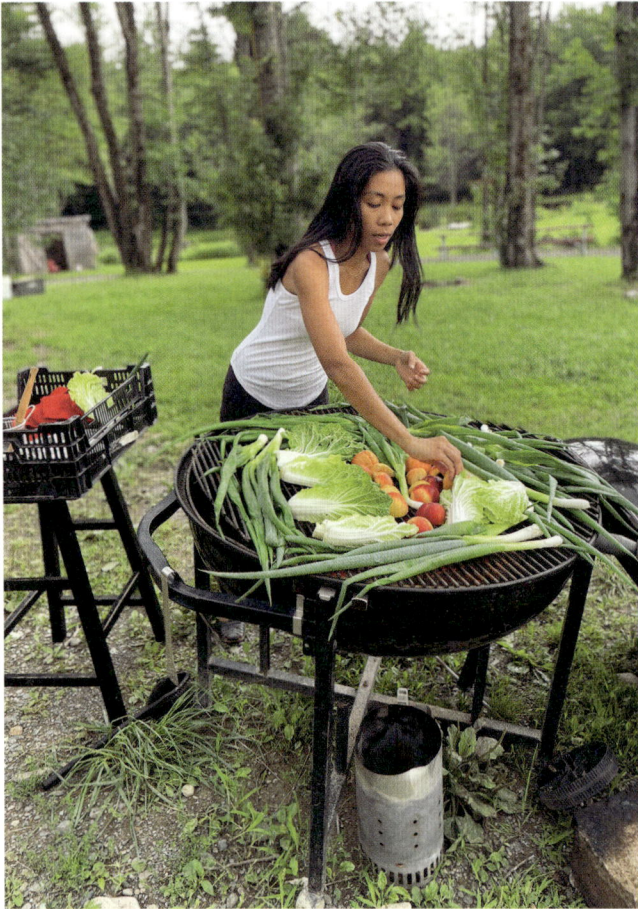

'We can't tell people they have to eat this apple if they think it's ugly, but if we make the ugly apple into an applesauce or apple bread, people will then eat it.'

The practice of nature

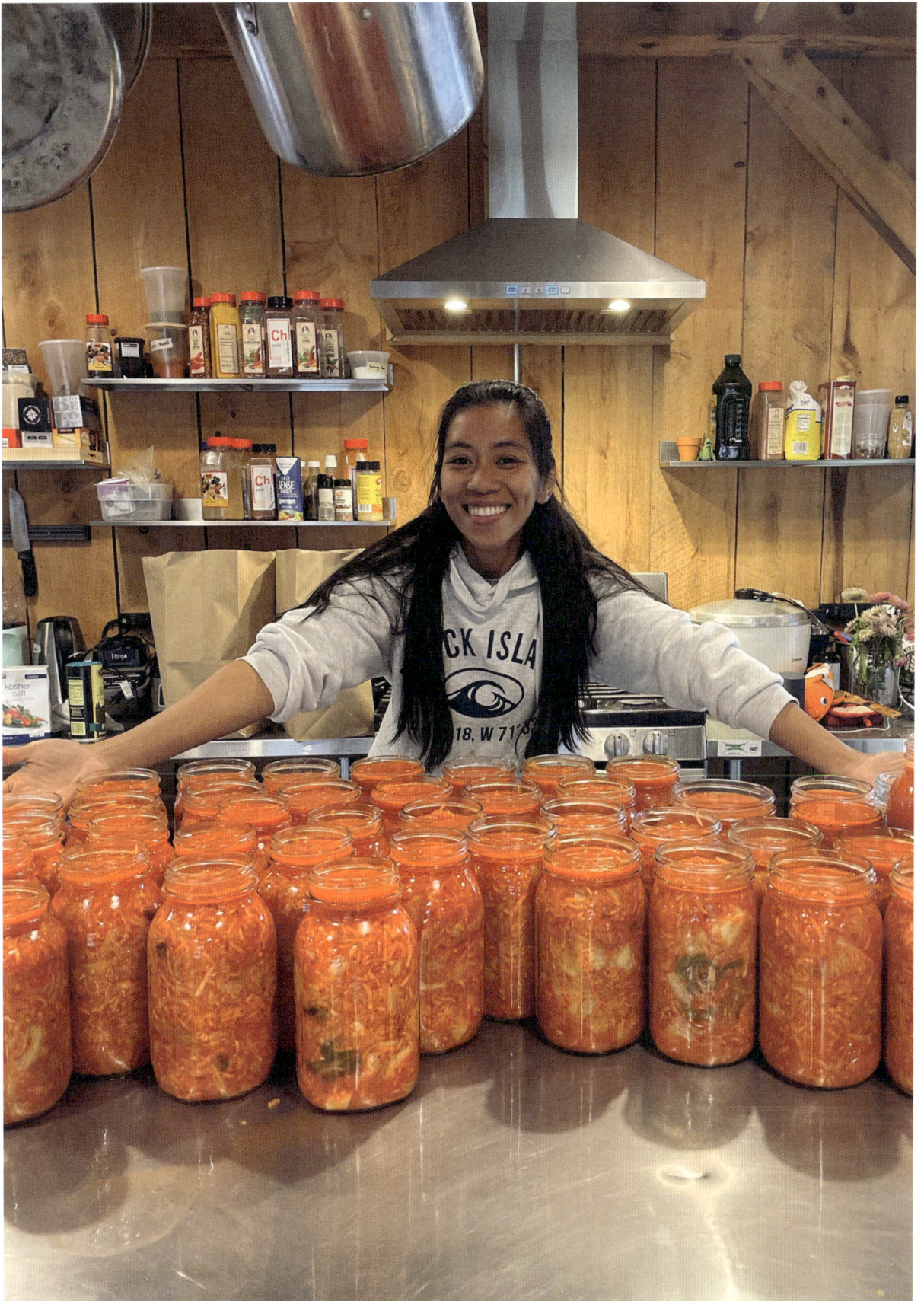

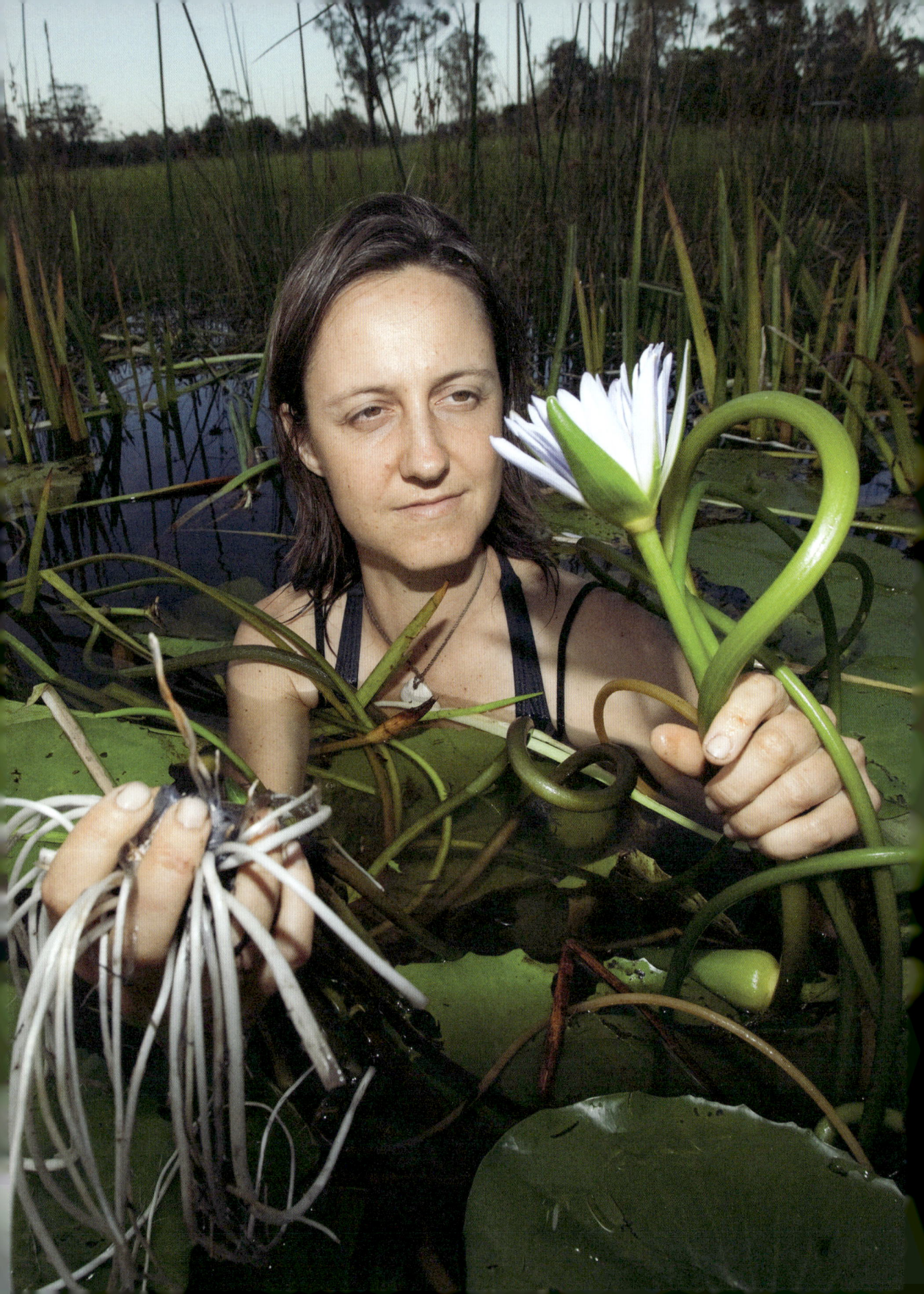

Wilderness immersion

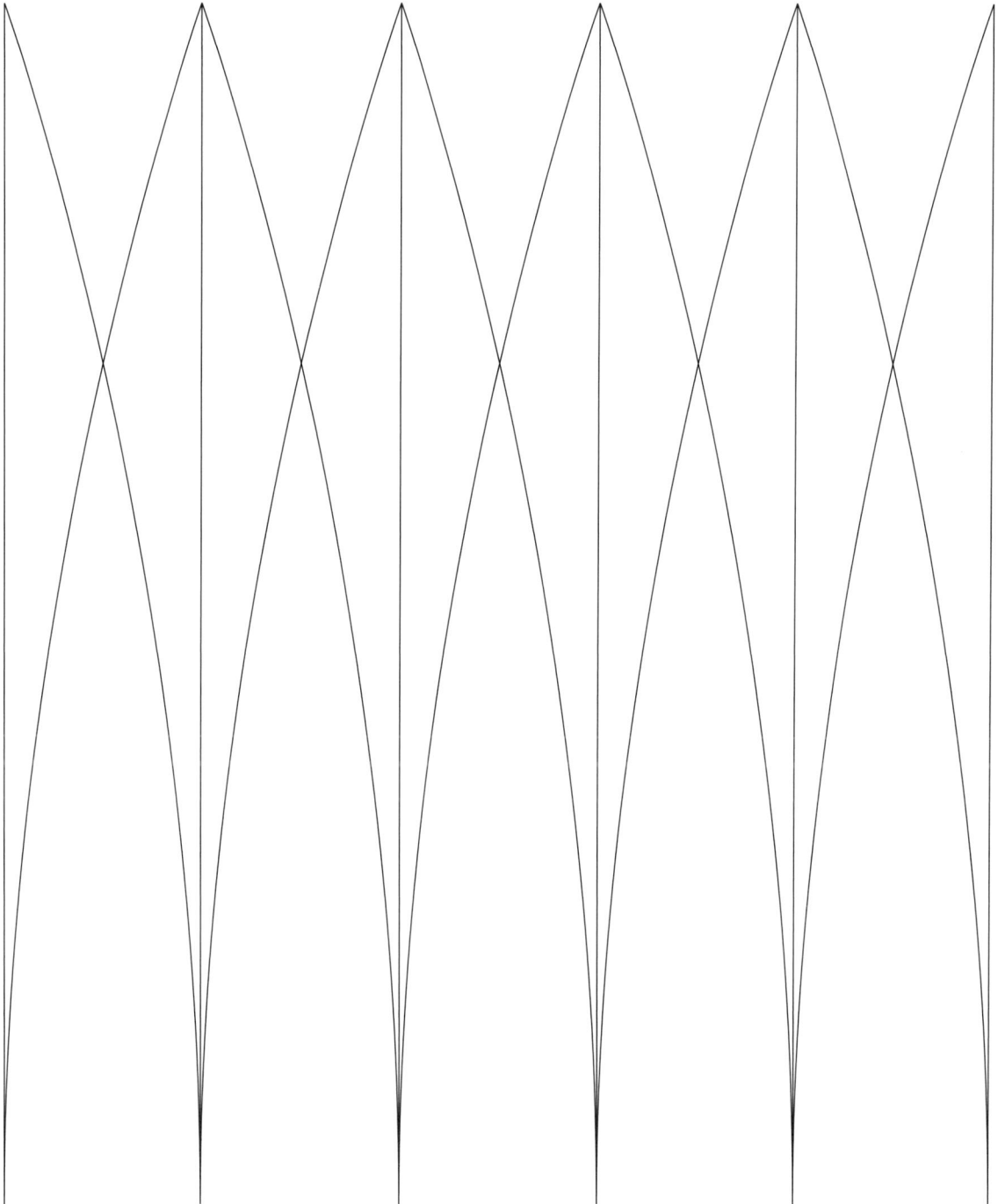

Facilitating personal growth in wild spaces

Claire Dunn

● Australia

After spending much of her twenties protesting to major corporations and the government, Claire Dunn made a bold move to live for a year in the bush off-grid. She built her own shelter, created fire from scratch (no lighters or matches), foraged food and practised bush crafts. Her journey took this new turn when she realised meaningful change could be made not from constantly defending nature but through building connections with it.

After spending twelve months in the wilderness, Claire had no idea that the return to normal life would prove to be one of the most profound lessons of all. She landed back in the concrete jungle of Melbourne, Australia, and formed a daily lifeline by finding the nearest green space. 'I need to be able to wander from home straight away into bush. I don't do very well in the suburbs. I feel very lucky to have found this place.' She refers to her home backing onto the Yarra River with tenderness and as a place that helped nurse the shock of returning to the city. It was also where she wrote her book *My Year Without Matches*.

After publishing the book, further self-enquiry and formal study in psychotherapy, Claire has morphed into a multi-modality practitioner. She blends facilitating nature connection workshops and contemporary wilderness rites of passage, mentoring and counselling clients in nature, teaching survival skills, and coaching people on ecological literacy. Summing it up as 'soul work', Claire describes her goal as helping people to realise their unique gifts and potential through the use of nature-based practices. 'It's really recognising that our relationship with "the wild other" and nature is integral to a life of connection and thriving. It is crucial that we remember ourselves as part of the living web of life.'

Claire has found that while the traditional wilderness and survival skills instructor roles tend to be held predominantly by men, the deep guided work of connecting with nature seems to be female dominated, and that goes for her participants too. 'There are some differences in the way that our cycles connect automatically to the cycles of Earth, the Sun and the Moon. We are more easily connected because we experience our own cycles every month, so there's a natural inclination there to want to dive deeper.'

While it's not in the wilderness or bush, Claire connects to nature on a daily basis in her garden. 'While simply tending the garden this year I've seen a tiger snake, a raptor that flies in and interacts with our chickens, and two hidden nests in the muddy banks belonging to spotted pardalotes (one of Australia's smallest birds). Gardening has the quality of both the wild and the cultivated, it's like a moving sit spot.'

Sit spots are an important part of Claire's daily life since learning the technique from a survival skills instructor many years ago. Claire explains, 'The sit spot is quite simply a place where one feels drawn to go regularly to sit in observation and in reverence to that environment. Mine is in my backyard but some people choose a park or other outdoor space they feel safe to sit in regardless of weather or time of day.'

Two of the most fundamental teachings from this and other practices in nature that Claire has engaged in are that 'the relationship of the inner landscape is interwoven with the outer landscape, and all is welcome – perfectionism really doesn't hold up in nature'.

The practice of nature

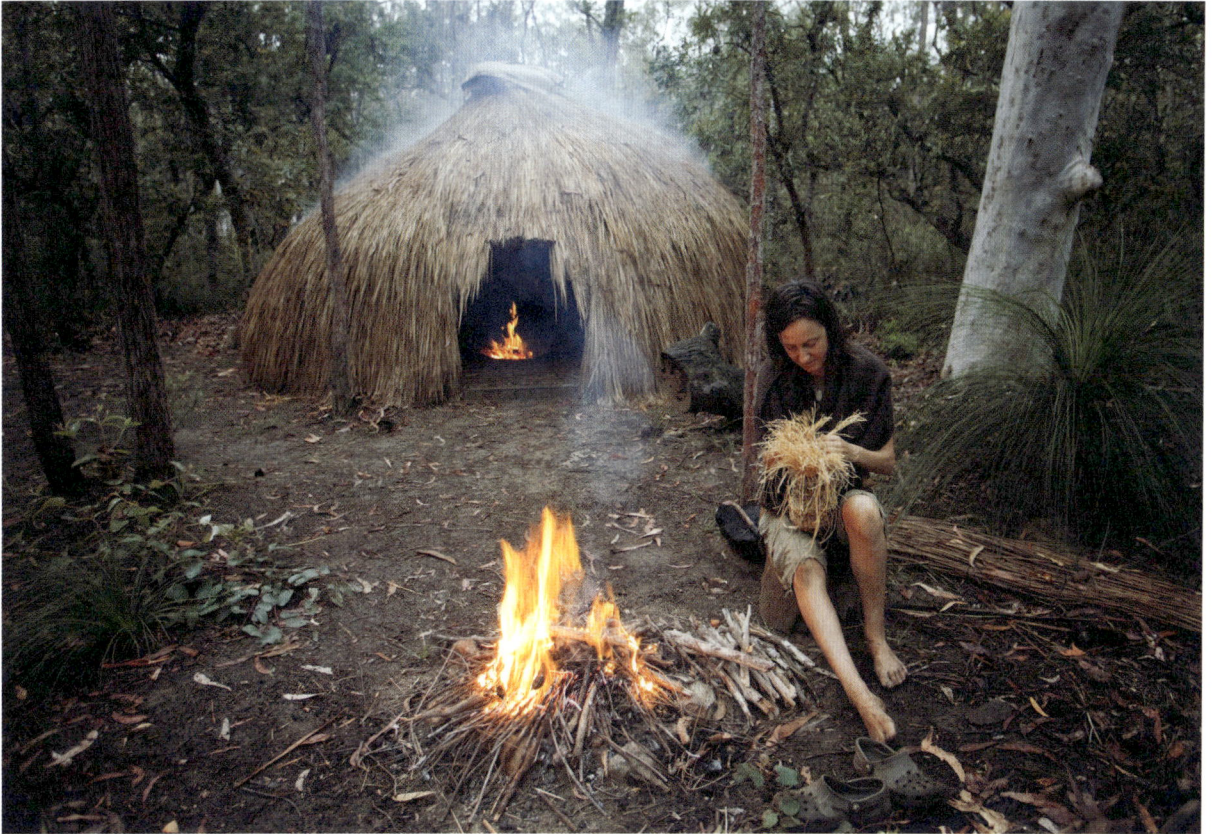

'What I came to understand was that the deeper cause of our ecological crisis was our Western culture's profound disconnection to the "more-than-human" world.'

Finding a sit spot to build a relationship with your local environment

Inspired by Claire Dunn

The purpose of a sit spot is to open your awareness to the happenings of an area and to notice the subtle beauties within nature. By cultivating a sit spot practice, you can become an expert in an area and come to understand the comings and goings of animals, the behaviour of plants according to the weather, and the changes in colours and textures and smells. It is essentially an awakening of the senses which can be beneficial in all facets of life.

There is emerging research investigating the benefits of 'grounding': the practice of standing or sitting directly on the earth. Scientists are exploring how our bodies can benefit from it with positive results reported on:

- lowered inflammation markers
- improved immune system responses
- reduced cardiovascular markers like respiratory rate and cortisol levels.

Taking the time to slow down and appreciate the pace of nature is vital for thriving in our fast-paced world. I'm often asking my patients to do less; to schedule downtime into their calendars and sit with the discomfort they may feel when not achieving anything. A practice such as a sit spot can be deeply nourishing for the nervous system, which then flows on to our digestion, our immune strength, our energy levels and our sleep quality.

To begin ●

● 1

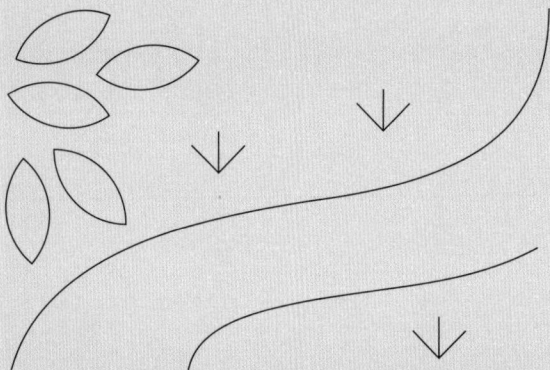

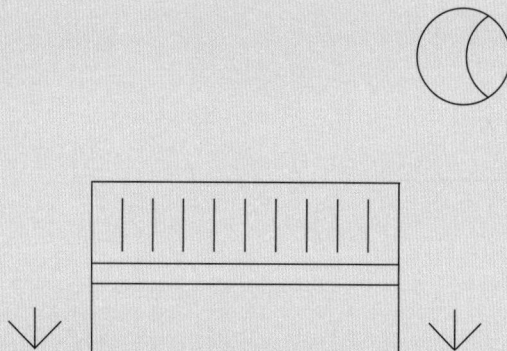

Find a place within a 5–10-minute walk from your home (your backyard is also fine) that has a wild quality and is safe to sit at all times of the day or night, weather and seasons.

● 2

Sit or lay still and quietly for as long as possible.

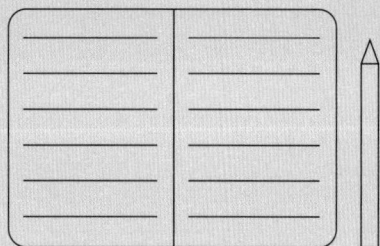

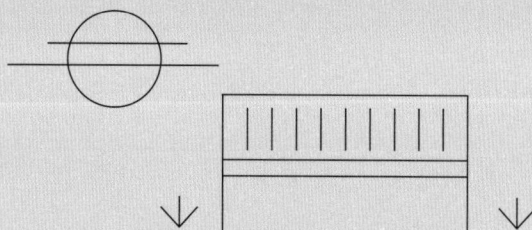

● 5

If you like to write, bring a notebook with you and reflect on your observations including how you felt and what you saw, smelt, touched and heard.

● 6

Go to this spot regularly to build your relationship with the area. If you can visit at different times of the day this can really enhance your experience of the place.

The practice of nature

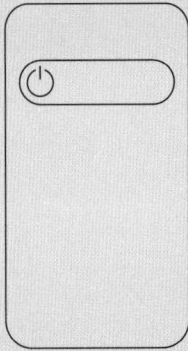

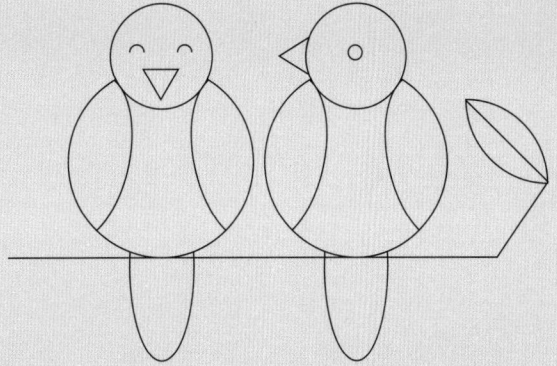

● 3
To stay present, leave your devices at home or switch them off while sitting in your spot.

● 4
Acutely observe what is going on in that small environment. Perhaps it is a family of birds that belong to a tree you sit underneath or a plant that is dancing in the wind.

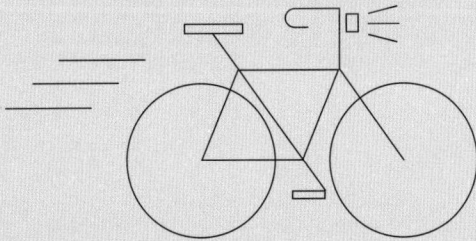

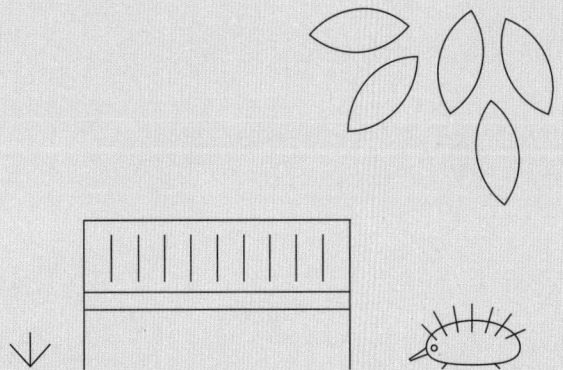

● 7
If you get a sense that this isn't the best spot for you, maybe there is noise from a nearby road or frequent disturbances from people walking by, find a new spot where you feel comfortable.

● 8
Stay curious about what you will see and learn because every day in nature is different to the next.

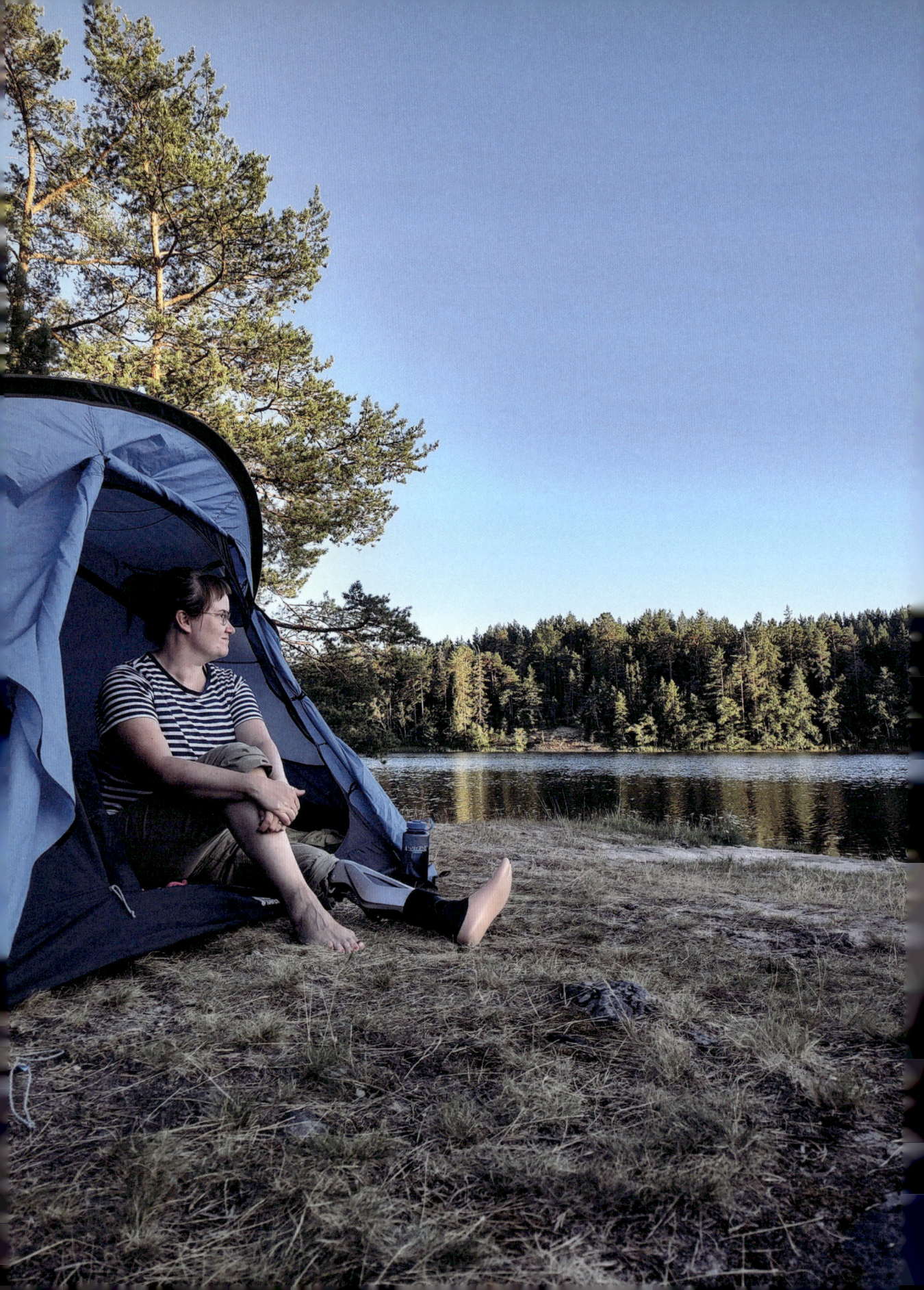

Hiking

Building confidence through hiking

Tiina
Nopanen

● Finland

'If I have worries
that I can't get over
in my head, I go
to nature. When
I come back my
worries are settled.'

At the age of fifteen, Tiina Nopanen had her left leg amputated above the knee after suffering from osteomyelitis (bone infection) since the age of four. While this was a difficult experience for any teenager to go through, she found that her time out in nature was personally healing. Nature is also a big part of the culture in her home country of Finland. The Finnish term *luontosuhde*, which translates to 'nature relationship', is something that most people in the country believe in, says Tiina. 'It's something that we get when we are born, we are raised to respect nature and go outdoors to hike as a family.'

Tiina says that hiking in Finland is taken quite seriously which can be difficult for her and others who can't always go great distances. 'People concentrate on how many kilometres you hike per day and that defines whether you are a real hiker or not. But I think it should be about spending time in nature. You can do so much more in nature other than just hiking.'

As a woman with an above-the-knee leg amputation, hiking long distances is not always possible or enjoyable. 'I prefer that the trail is a bit flatter and easier so that I can look at the scenery, otherwise I just have to look down at the tree roots and rocks and where I place my feet so I don't fall,' says Tiina, highlighting one of the biggest challenges amputees experience with hiking. This is a key reason why Tiina decided to start her Instagram page. 'I want to show that there are so many more people going outdoors. In social media and marketing for outdoor clothing brands, they give us this image that the only people who go outdoors are white, slim and able-bodied.'

With this in mind, Tiina recently spent time presenting at a fair in Helsinki in collaboration with the Paralympic Committee to highlight the different ways that people with disabilities can access nature. She is also currently working with the company who made her prosthetic leg to plan a hiking event for amputees. 'The biggest obstacles are in our own minds, we just have to go out and try, that is the main thing. If you believe you can't, then you won't be able to do it. You can still do things but maybe you do it differently to an able-bodied person,' she says.

Tiina remembers how she felt when she was finally able to go on her first longer distance hike and wants that for others too. 'It was a big step to go on my first real hike which was 10 kilometres in the north of Finland. It gave me a feeling of overcoming myself. I managed to do this,' she reflects. Hiking has also advanced Tiina's fitness and improved her balance, something vital for an amputee to feel more confident.

Along with these personal gains, Tiina and her husband of twenty years will frequently go out to experience nature together. One of their favourite things to do is to rent an off-the-grid cabin where they have to collect their water from the lake and cook food by the fire. She says these trips help them to go back to their roots and slow down. In the winter when there is too much soft snow, making it difficult for Tiina to hike, she will bring nature inside by going through photographs her husband has taken on their hiking trips or admire things she has brought inside. 'In Finland we have this thing where you take a match box and you put some rocks, moss or grass in it and carry it in your pocket. Whenever you want to feel like you are outdoors, you can smell it or feel it and get the sense of nature wherever you are.'

Tiina wants to highlight that nature can be part of everyone's life. She is hopeful that Finland and other places around the world will continue to develop accessible hiking trails so that no matter your ability, you can get outdoors. Her advice for anyone who is starting out, or who may have never gone hiking before, is to just give it a go.

'Go outside and try, you don't have to start hard and go on a long hike. Start easy and when you feel you can manage that, increase the difficulty little by little. If you start too hard it might be a letdown. Even just spending time in nature will give you benefits; you don't always have to hike.'

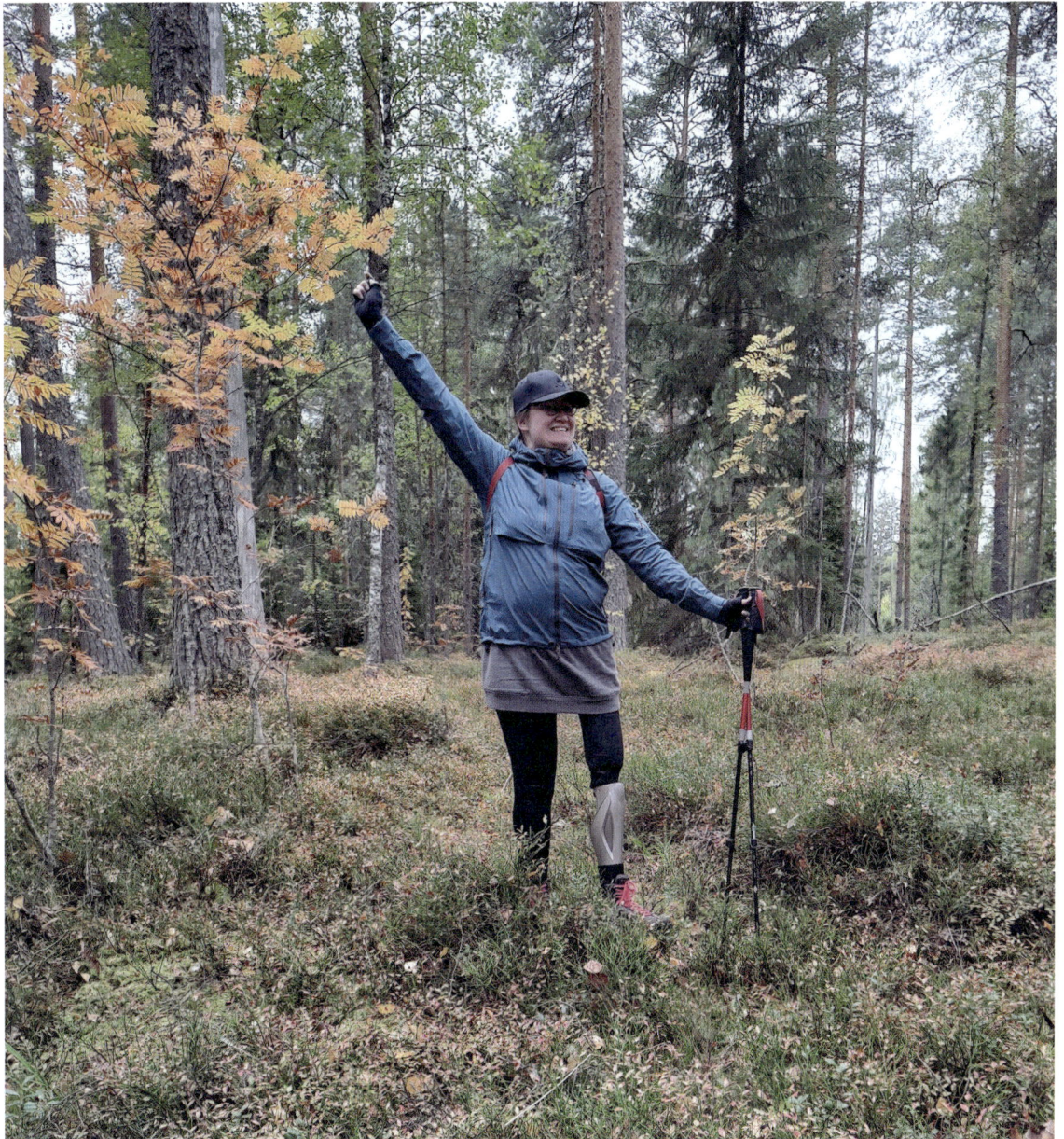

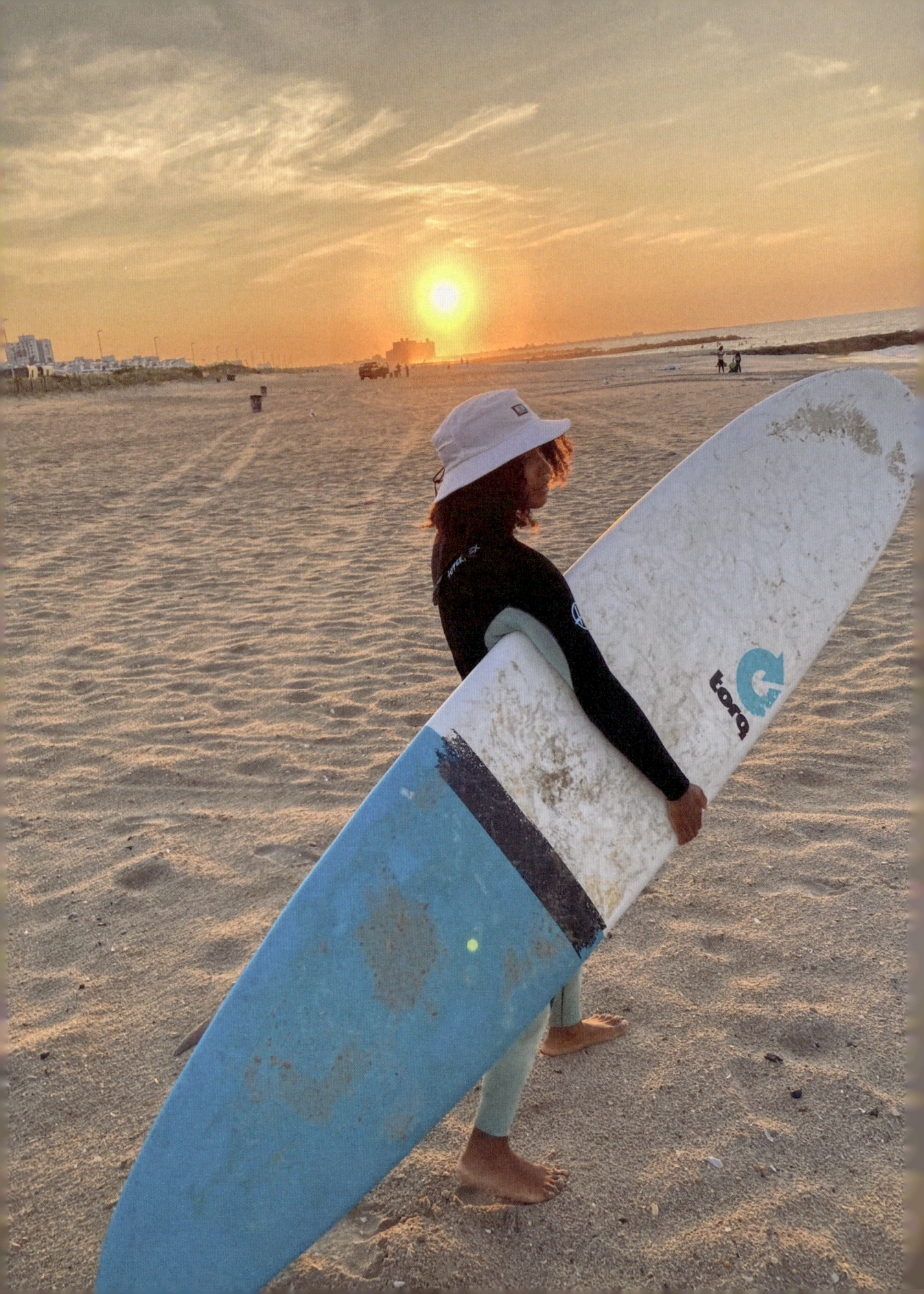

Surfing

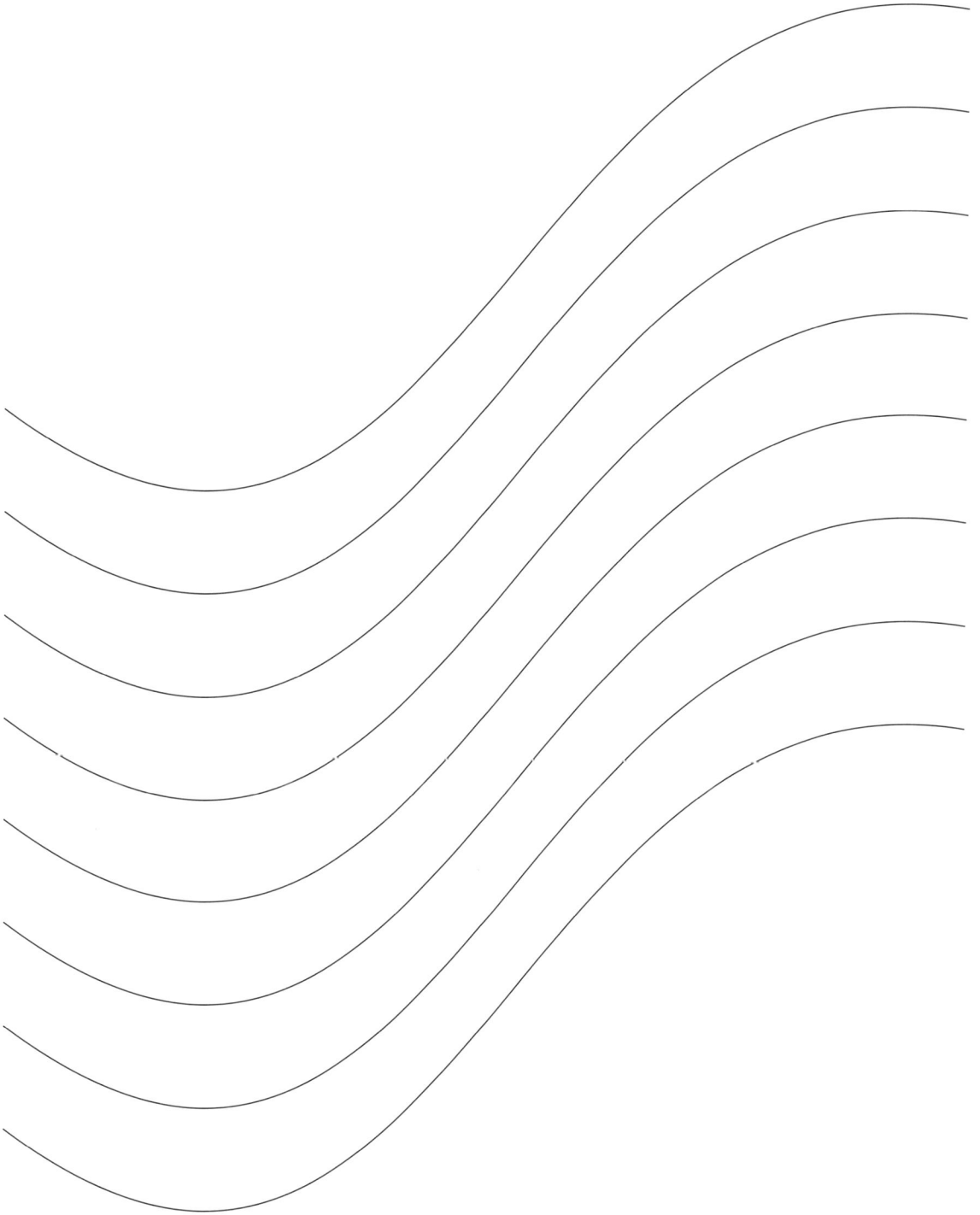

Breaking stereotypes in the surf

Autumn
Kitchens

● USA

When Autumn Kitchens went for her first surf lesson on the beaches of Long Island, New York, USA, she instantly fell in love. Ten years later and surfing is now the centre of her life. Working as a surf instructor and at a surfing not-for-profit called Laru Beya Collective, Autumn is following a path that she never thought she would. 'I'm supposed to be a midwife right now. As a slight perfectionist I think, "this is not where I should be, this is not what I thought I would be doing at twenty-four years old", but for the past year I've been learning I'm in no rush. I'm enjoying the present and surrendering to that idea.'

For Autumn, midwifery and surf instructing are, in a way, comparable. Both roles support and encourage people to step into their own power and help to build courage through a new experience. Autumn says, 'If you can be comfortable in the ocean, there is a level of confidence that you carry with you everywhere you go.' And this is part of the reason why she loves to work with children. 'I've seen a child go from not even wanting to put their toe in the ocean to jumping off a surfboard into green waves. To see that progression in someone is inspiring.'

'Seeing children not only become comfortable in the ocean but learn how to surf and grow their joy for it is life changing. The ocean is so impactful, the children's minds are growing and processing right in front of you.'

It's not only children that Autumn wants to get into the ocean, but also other minorities in the surf world. 'Black and brown communities have been taught that they don't belong in the water. So, we need to convince them that messaging isn't true.' Growing up, seeing other people of colour in the surf was a rarity for Autumn. 'I never surfed with people that looked like me until last summer. So it's something that I'm working on with other people,' she says. While there might not be any official statistics on how many surfers are Caucasian compared to people of colour, it is safe to say that white people appear to make up the majority – and white men at that.

Thankfully, Autumn has already seen a shift in gender dynamics in the surf. 'There are a lot more women in the surf now compared to when I was growing up. In the summer there are so many women, sometimes there are more women than men,' she says excitedly. The reason why this change is important to Autumn is because it allows her to feel safer and freer in the ocean. 'I look very young and I'm quite small, so men have automatically assumed that I don't know what I'm doing,' she says. 'There's a feeling that I have to be perfect in the water, I can't make any mistakes and give them a reason to make comments.' This feeling of perfectionism took a lot of the play out of surfing for Autumn. When she gets to surf with other women, she feels she can let go and have more fun.

Outside of having fun and opening opportunities for other people to enjoy the ocean, Autumn finds surfing to be deeply medicinal. 'I can be an overthinker and an anxious person, so to have something that keeps me present is very important.' When going into the ocean, Autumn says she feels at one with Earth. 'It's incredibly grounding but at the same time exhilarating. I don't think there are lots of things you can do to have both of those feelings in one.' Using nature as a form of self-love, a panacea for one's biggest struggles, is something Autumn wishes to be known for.

As someone who grew up in New York, all of Autumn's fondest memories of time spent in nature are at the beach. She acknowledges that she is privileged to live both close to the ocean and to have found her true passion in life and she wishes the same for everyone. 'If there is ever a thought to experience the ocean, experience surfing, experience nature in whatever medium, do it! That thought is there for a reason.'

'Surfing teaches us that there will always be moments of frustration but whatever is meant to be will be – your wave will come.'

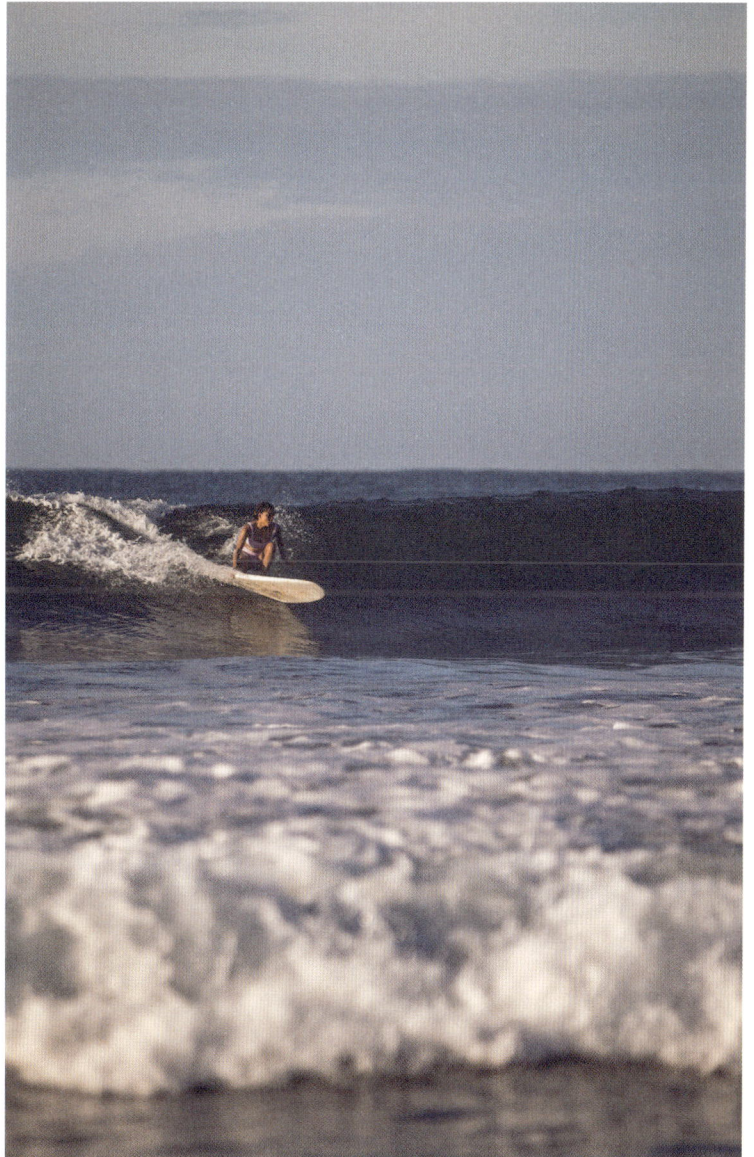

'Nature in general
is so healing,
especially the
ocean. As women,
our bodies are in
sync with nature;
with the tides.'

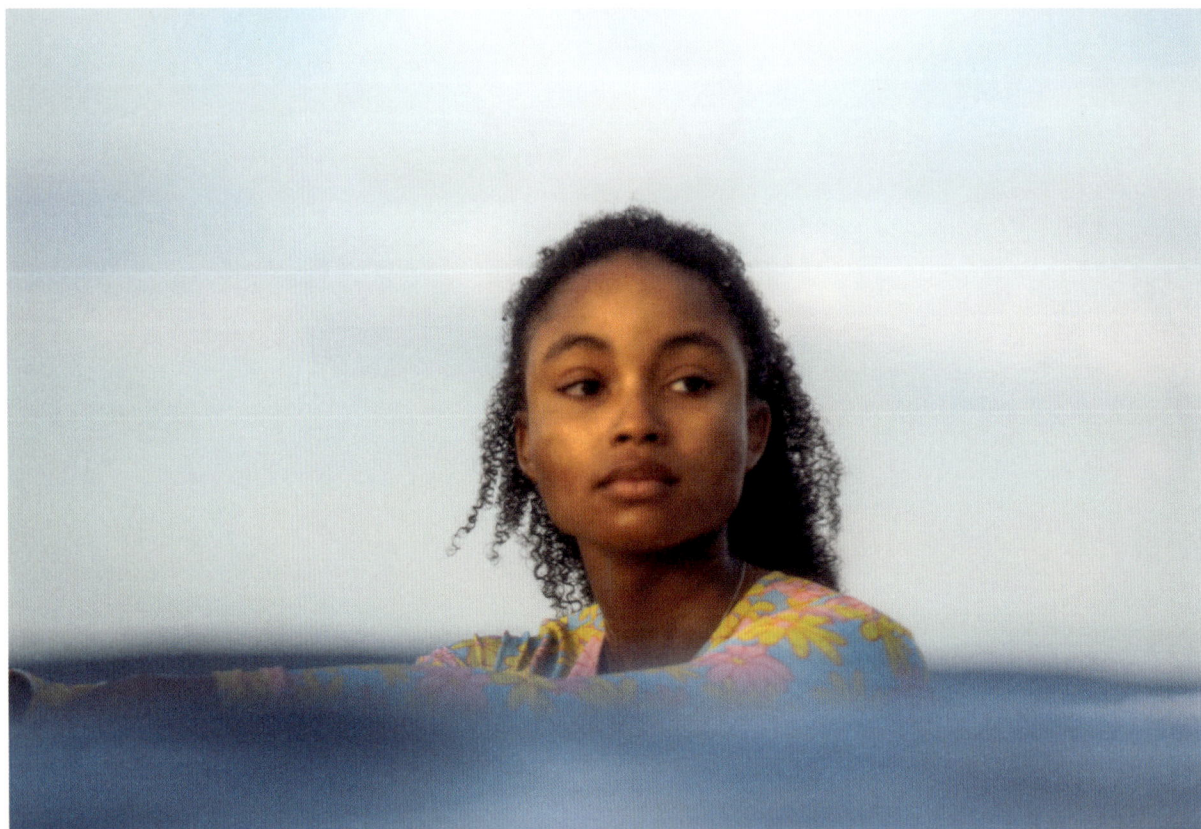

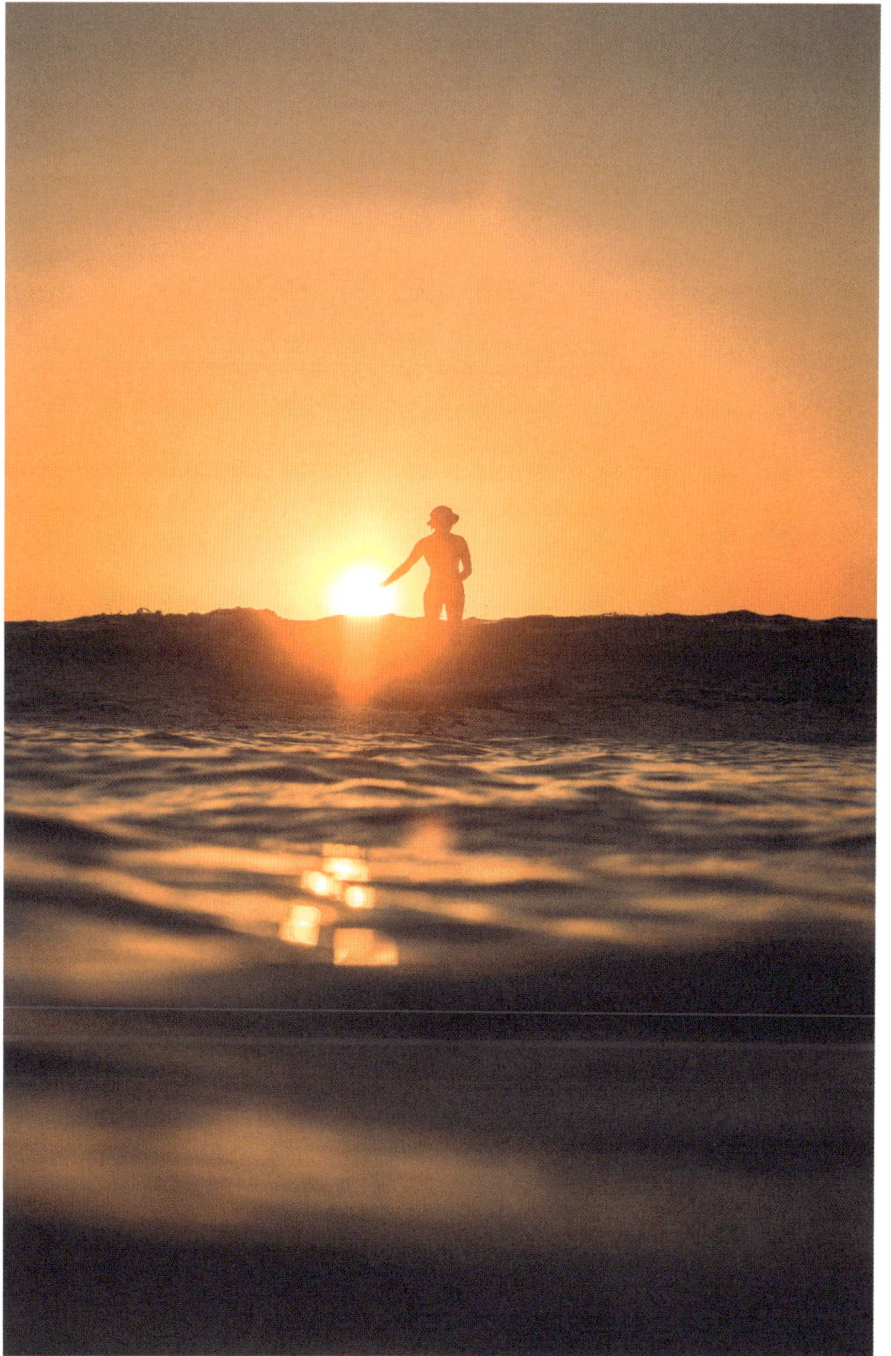

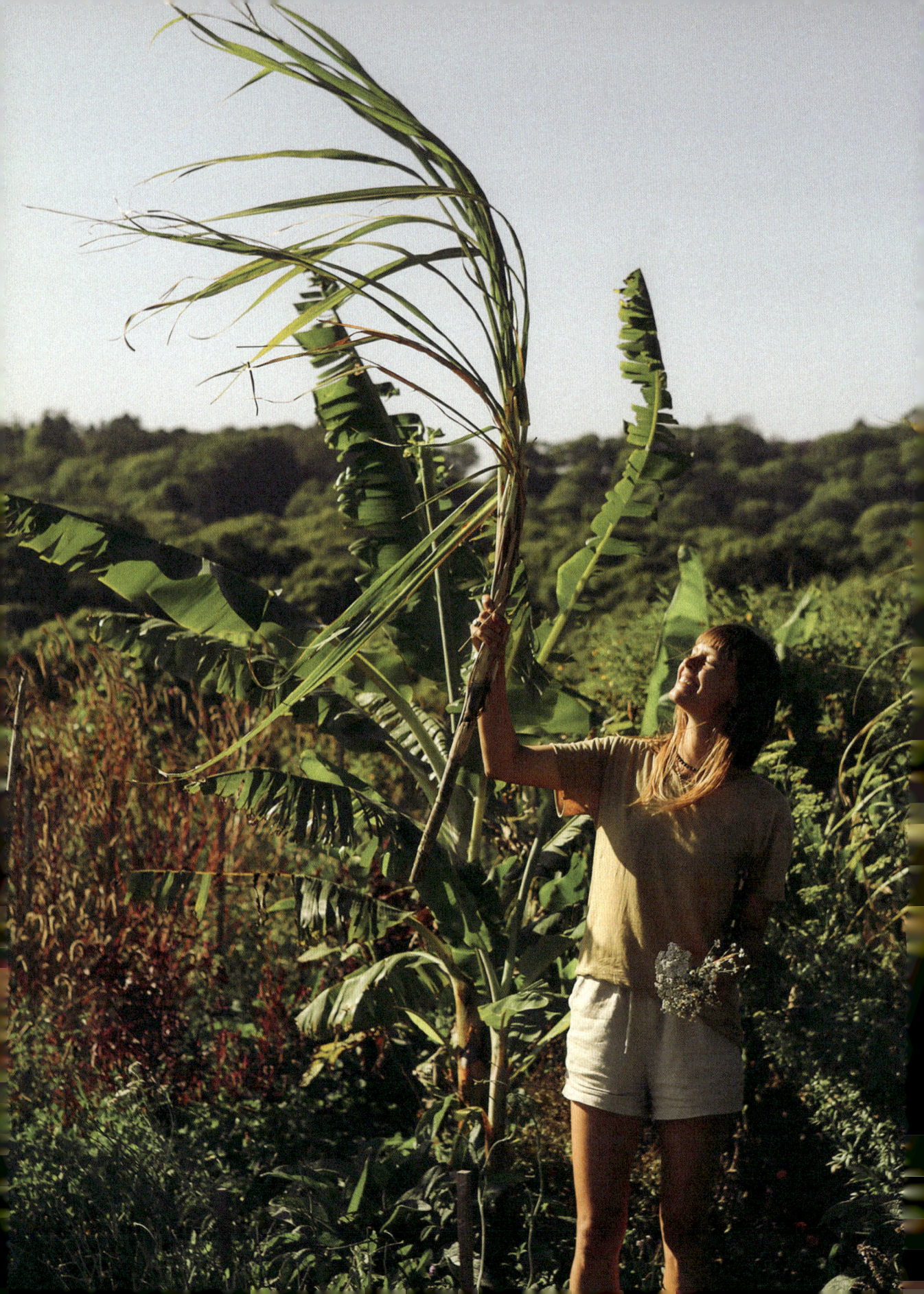

Permaculture

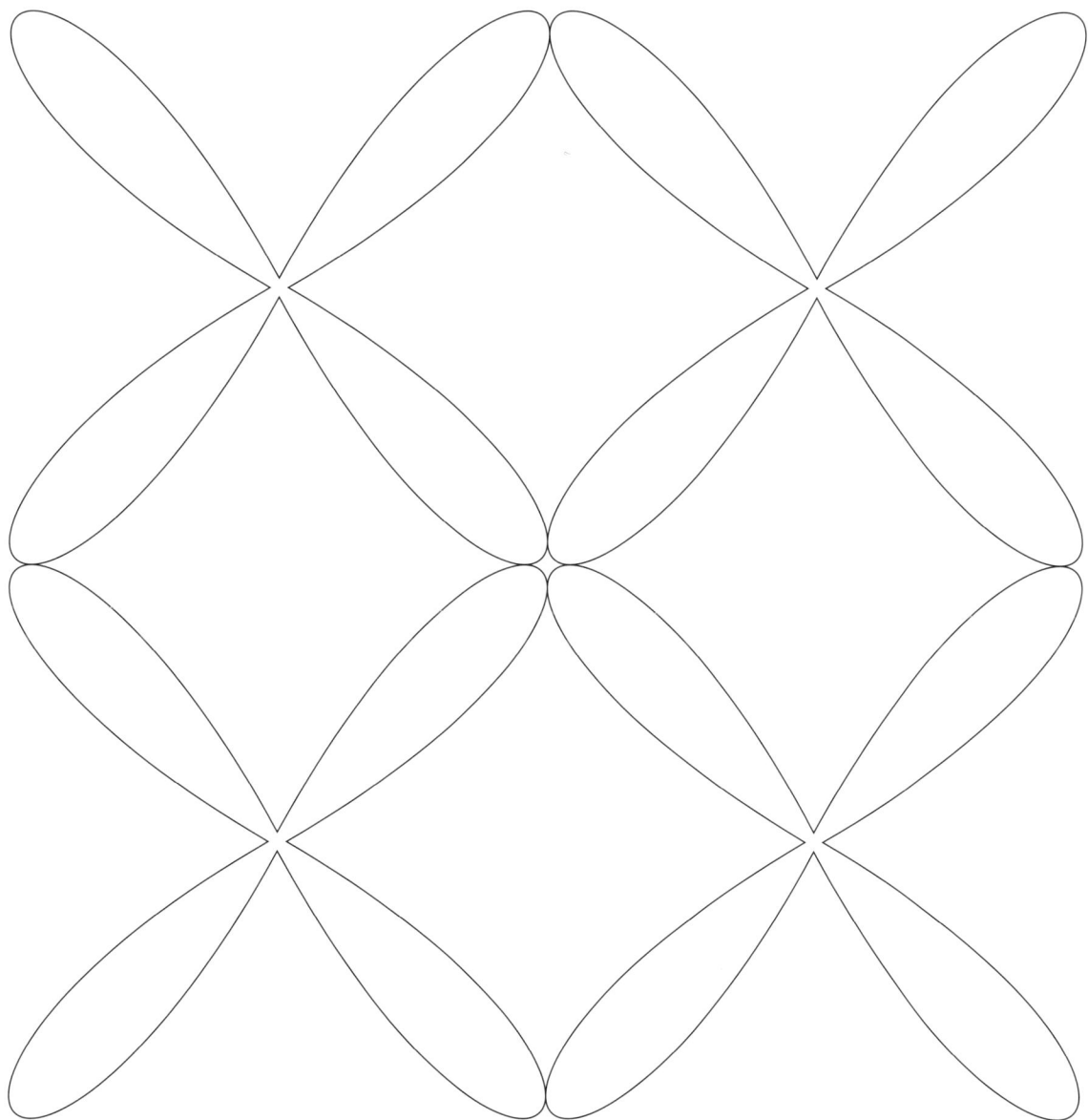

Using gardening to create community

Kobi Bloom

● Australia

After spending years in Sydney, Australia, as a young adult exploring her creativity and enjoying the social aspects of a big city, Kobi Bloom evolved into a different stage of life. She wanted to focus on connecting more with the land and plants to forge a new path: a life of permaculture.

'People see permaculture as a bit of a hippy-dippy messy backyard but it's pretty complex and I think every single aspect of life can be practised with permaculture in mind,' she says. Kobi explains how the principles of permaculture really just imply a permanent culture; one that is sustainable and can continue on. 'It's about working with nature, not just taking from nature, to create a sustainable lifestyle, including feeding, clothing and sheltering ourselves.'

Often compared to landscaping, which, in essence, is mostly about aesthetics, permaculture requires many layers designed for function. It is a reciprocity between different plants, the soil and the local wildlife. 'Generally, horticulture and landscaping is about creating order and having clear spaces, but in terms of the way nature works, there needs to be that biodiversity – that jungle element.' The reciprocity between plants and soil is comparable to the way Kobi works within her local community, exchanging information and sharing skills for the enhancement of the collective.

'Plants communicate and share with each other, they share carbon, water and information. Plants in pots can't do that. It's quite symbolic, it translates back to the way we live. Plants are incredibly resilient, but they won't have the same nutrient quality as if they were connected to the soil and it's exactly the same as humans. If humans are isolated, they can survive, but there is something missing.'

Since moving to the Byron Bay region in Australia, being part of the community has been an integral part of Kobi's life. She runs regular workshops around the local area to encourage and educate others to engage with the natural environment as much as possible, as well as to form bonds with people. 'One of the biggest motivators for me to keep doing what I'm doing is to be surrounded by other people who are interested in the same thing. When those people aren't in your life it makes it very difficult. We are not islands; we don't operate that way. I don't think many people are inspired or motivated to do things just for themselves with no one else around who understands or acknowledges it.'

Kobi describes that her favourite way of connecting with nature is to eat it – particularly the things most of us would throw away. Weeds in particular are one of Kobi's true loves. Labelling them as 'feral food', she will pick weeds every day to include in her diet. Kobi wants to encourage a change of mindset around certain plants that are usually sprayed and pulled out. 'Everyone can access them; it's food for the people. To me weeds represent rebellious people. Foraging for weeds is very cool, it's one of the most rebellious things we can do.' Kobi acknowledges that we have become sensitised to certain flavours like bitter or sour, which are found in these types of plants, but the nutritional and medicinal qualities for her far outweigh the taste.

In her work, Kobi feels a great deal of pressure around ensuring she is offering the best information and doing the right thing for future generations. Many of her workshops cater to children, which she says gives her a sense of contribution and feeling as though she is doing something positive for the world. 'Working with kids is one of the most rewarding experiences for me because they are so close to nature. Even if they have grown up in an apartment, you can take them back into a space where you are helping them focus their attention on nature again and it happens just like that.'

Children, Kobi says, are much more in tune and connect with nature easily, and this can often be the gateway for building and strengthening communities. This is why Kobi continues to offer these classes, connecting as many people as possible to the land. 'There is awe and wonder; that is the part of humans that gets a little bit dampened and hidden over the years as we grow up and we have responsibilities. But that wonder is one of the biggest change makers.'

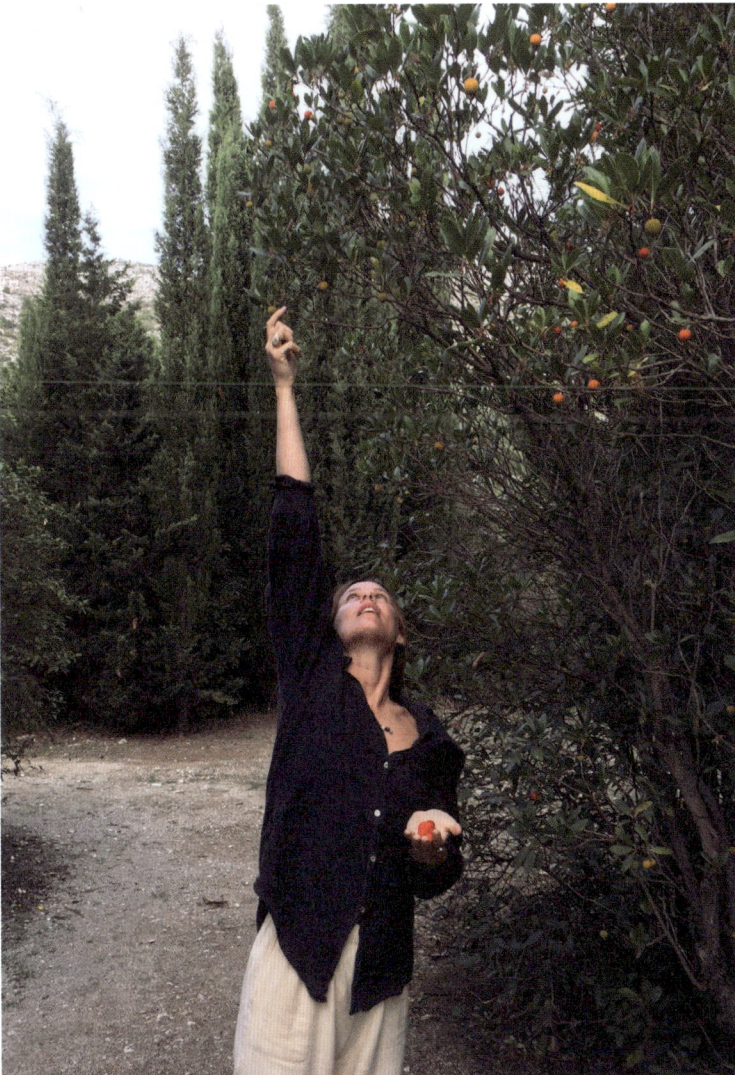

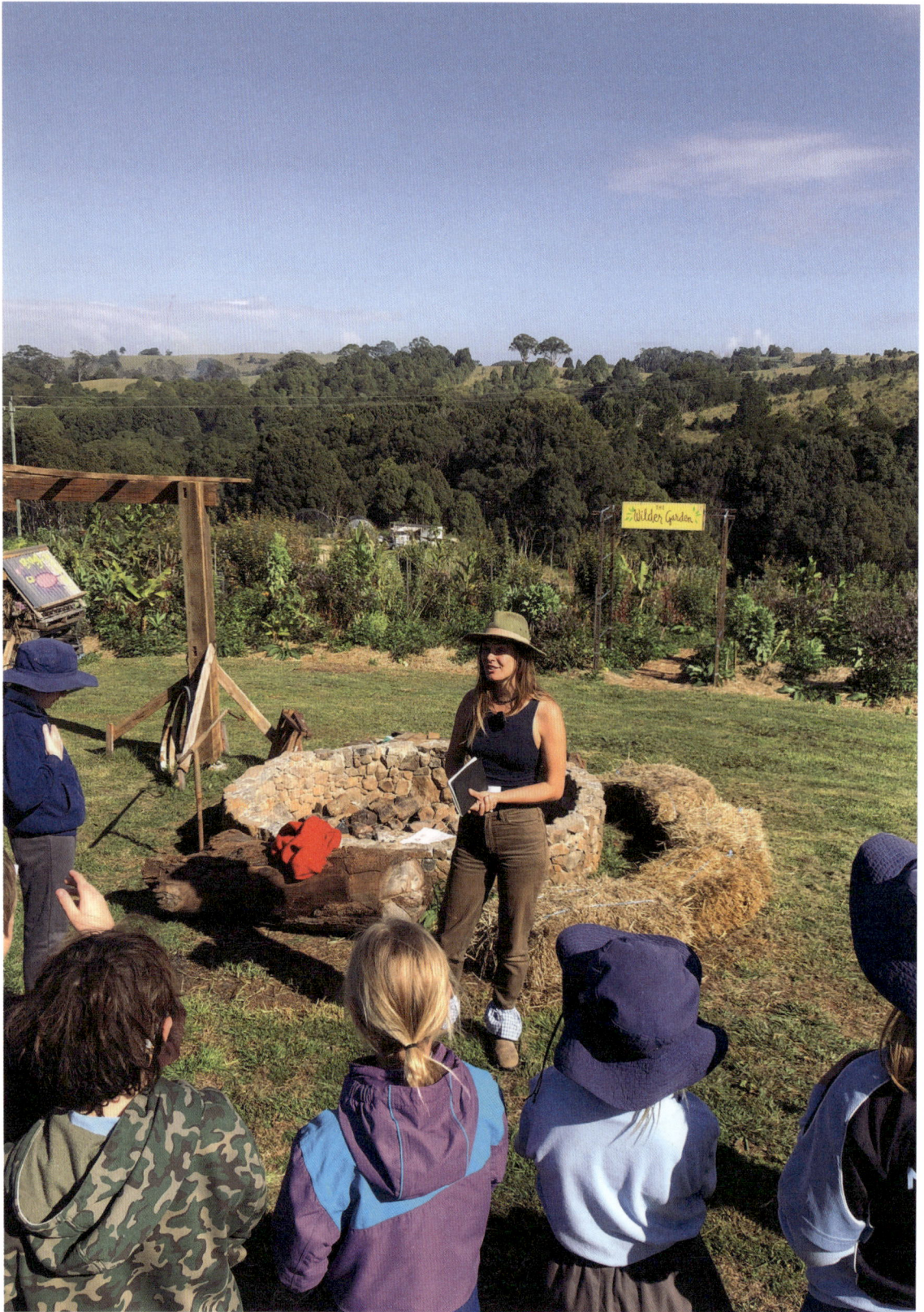

The practice of nature

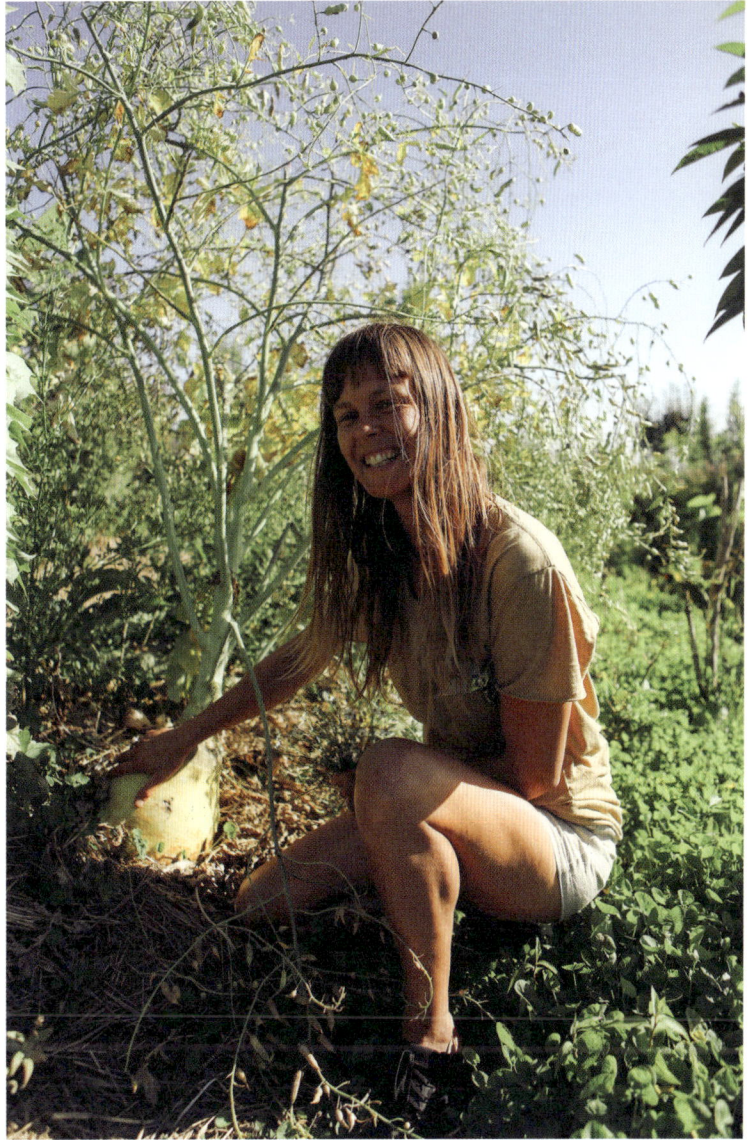

'It's about working
with nature, not
just taking from
nature, to create a
sustainable lifestyle.'

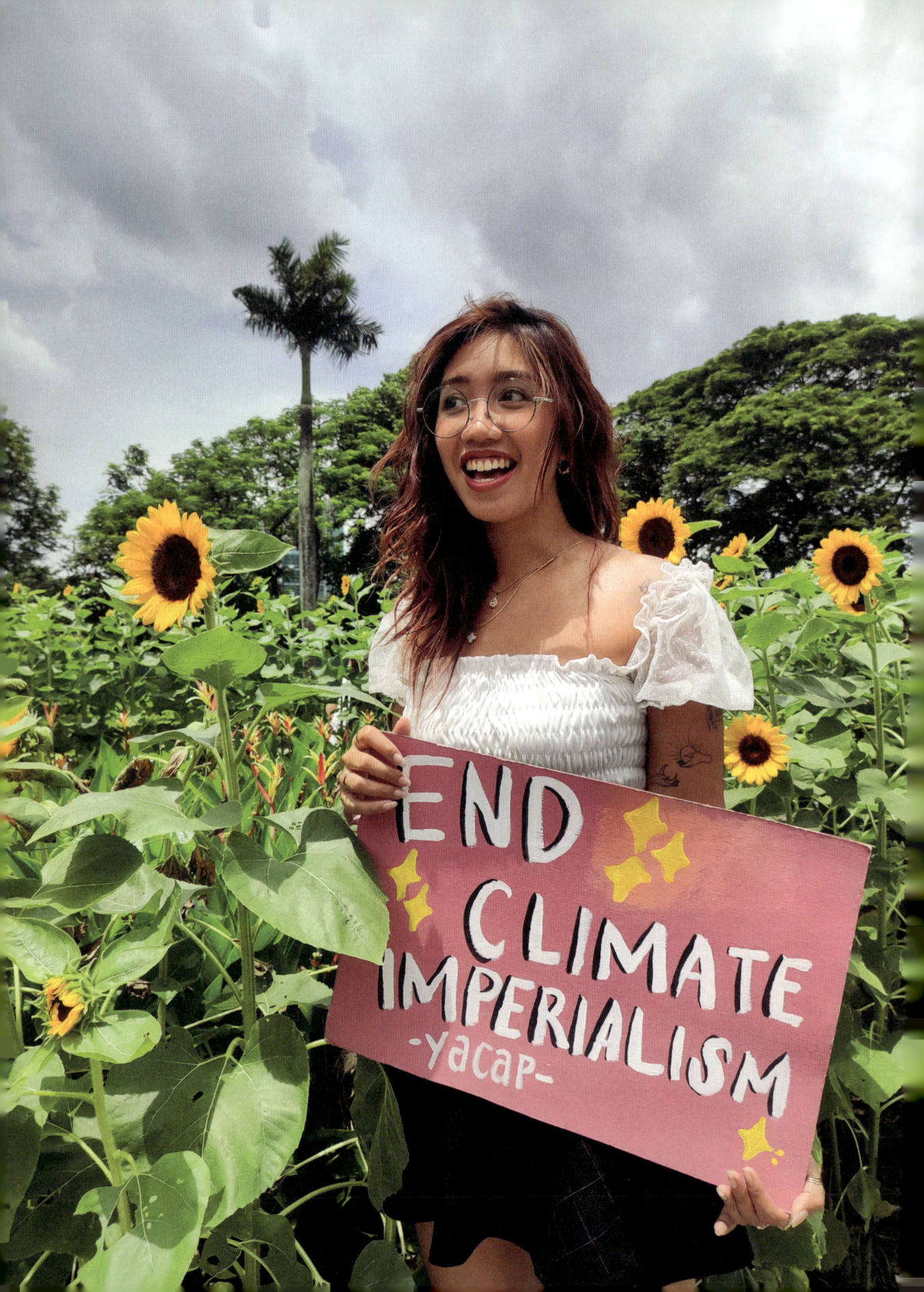

Climate activism

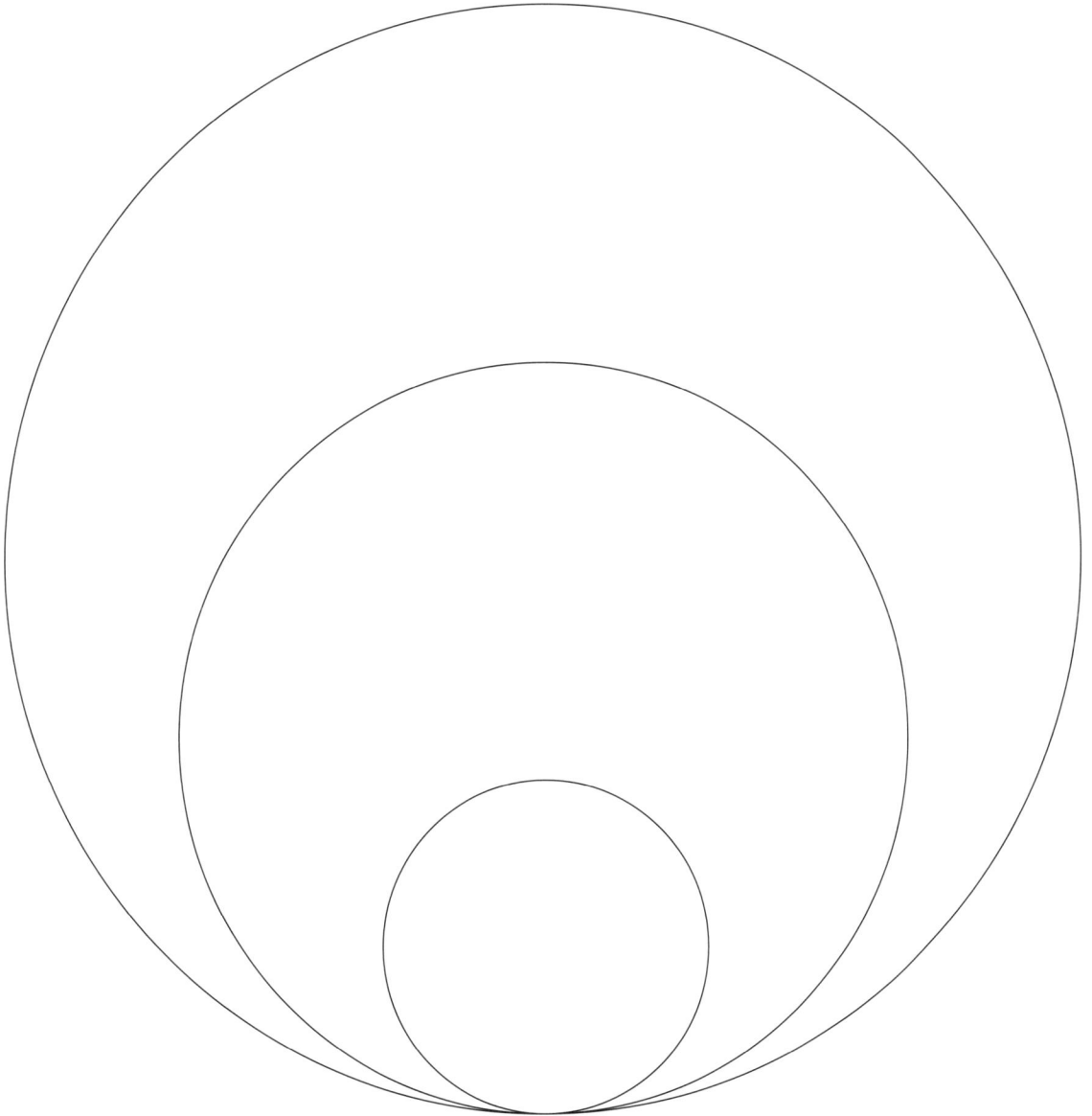

Advocating for change for future generations

Mitzi Jonelle Tan

● Philippines

'The system that we are in looks at everything as a natural resource to use rather than something we are part of. People are a part of nature too.'

Mitzi Jonelle Tan from Manila, in the Philippines, has always had a strong reaction to environmental changes. She remembers as a child being stuck inside for days due to flooding from a typhoon. When she went outside to get food, all the trees she grew up with had been uprooted and she began to cry. 'My parents were wondering if there was something wrong and I said that Earth was hurt. Even at that young age they said that I saw and recognised what was happening.' The image of the flooding stuck with Mitzi and fuelled her passion for advocating towards climate justice many years later.

Mitzi didn't join the climate justice movement full-time until she had the opportunity to meet with a group of Lumad Indigenous people. One of the leaders told her that 'they were not climate activists; they just had no choice but to fight back'. A simple sentence that completely changed Mitzi's trajectory. 'I realised he was right. Who was I to have all these privileges – an education and stable income – but I was choosing when it was convenient for me to fight when there are people who have no choice but to fight back constantly?'

Communities, such as the Lumad people, rely heavily on their local flora and fauna to sustain them for their food and materials. In turn they have a deep reverence for what the environment provides for them. 'Farmers and fisherfolk don't call themselves climate activists or environmental defenders. They don't do it to save the environment, they do it because they are part of the environment. They know that they are co-dependent with the environment, with nature.'

Coming from a fishing family, Mitzi's grandfather moved to Manila with his wife for better opportunities. They were inspired by the Lapu-Lapu statue in the centre of the city, a monument that represents anti-colonial resistance, and began taking photographs there every year on Christmas morning. 'It's something that the family has passed on, but in thirty years that area is going to be flooded, it will be below sea level. That generational tradition will probably end with me or my children,' says Mitzi with a heavy sadness.

Mitzi's parents have personally witnessed the impacts of climate change. 'When I talk to my mum, she tells me that it wasn't like this when she was growing up. Yes, the Philippines has always been prone to typhoons, but it wasn't this intense. It wasn't this frequent.' One of the more concerning parts for Mitzi is that after all these decades of climate change, the Philippines still doesn't have adequate evacuation protocols in place. 'Evacuation centres are schools and gyms which also flood and break because they are not climate-resilient infrastructures. Even when the typhoon is gone, people are stuck in schools because they can't go home yet and children's education suffers because of that.'

As with many people who are deeply passionate about a social movement, Mitzi initially found it difficult to relate to friends and family who weren't also getting involved with activism. However, over time she has changed tactics to lead by example rather than force; as for some people, seeing a person they know care about something deeply can often make them care about it more.

For the people who do want to get involved, Mitzi says you don't have to quit your day job to become an activist. 'I think every single

The practice of nature

person has their role in the movement and they don't have to radically change what they are doing or themselves to be able to do that. If you write policy, that is activism. If you are an accountant that helps an activist, that also contributes.' Simply educating yourself and making choices that reflect your beliefs can be a stance for climate justice.

It can be dangerous being a climate activist in the Philippines and it comes with many risks. The organisations that Mitzi works with need to have certain safety measures in place for all of their members. Despite this, Mitzi says that while she is safe, she will continue protesting, speaking and sharing. 'The more people that are talking about it, the safer it becomes for people who constantly talk about it. They can't arrest everyone right?' This sense of optimism is part of Mitzi's strategy. She does not want to be an angry activist; she wants to be loving and gentle. 'A lot of my anger and fear and sadness stems from a place of love, love for the people, the planet and for life. That gives me so much hope.'

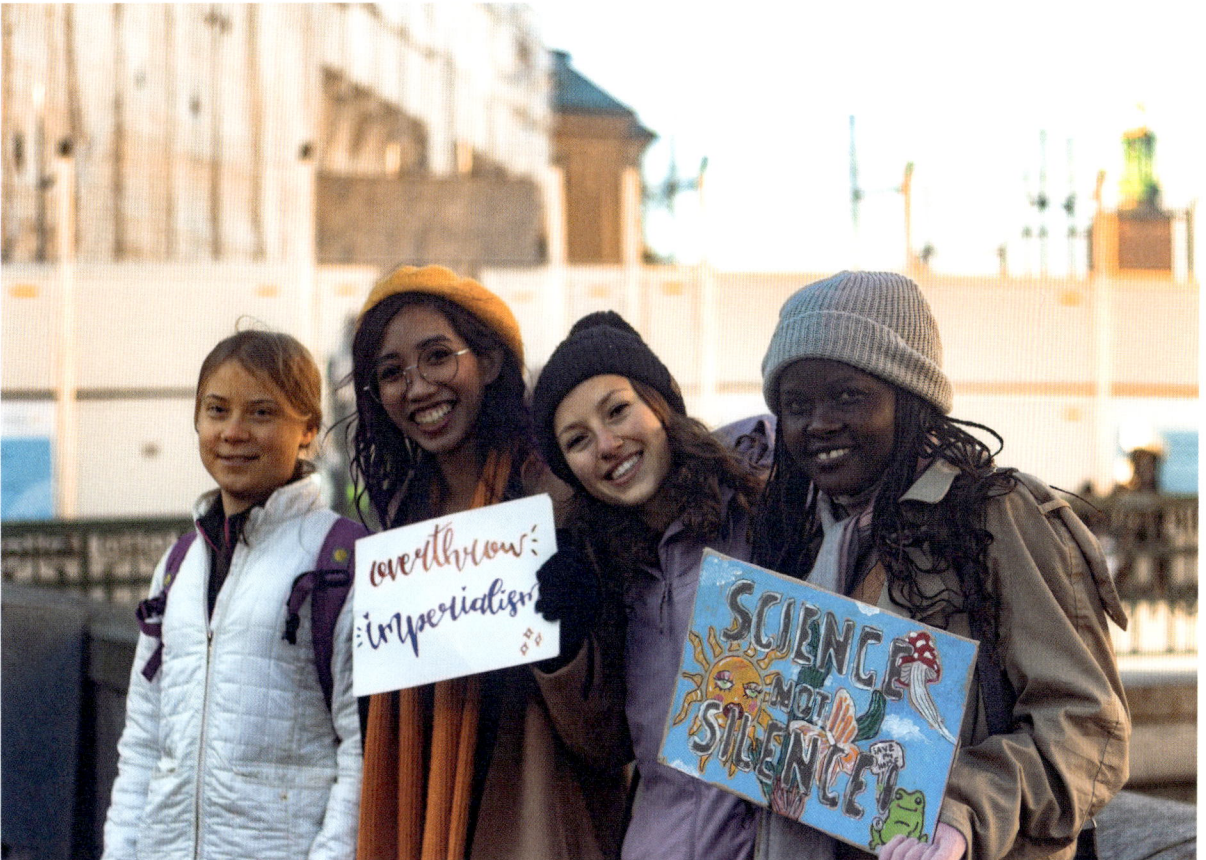

The wisdom
of nature

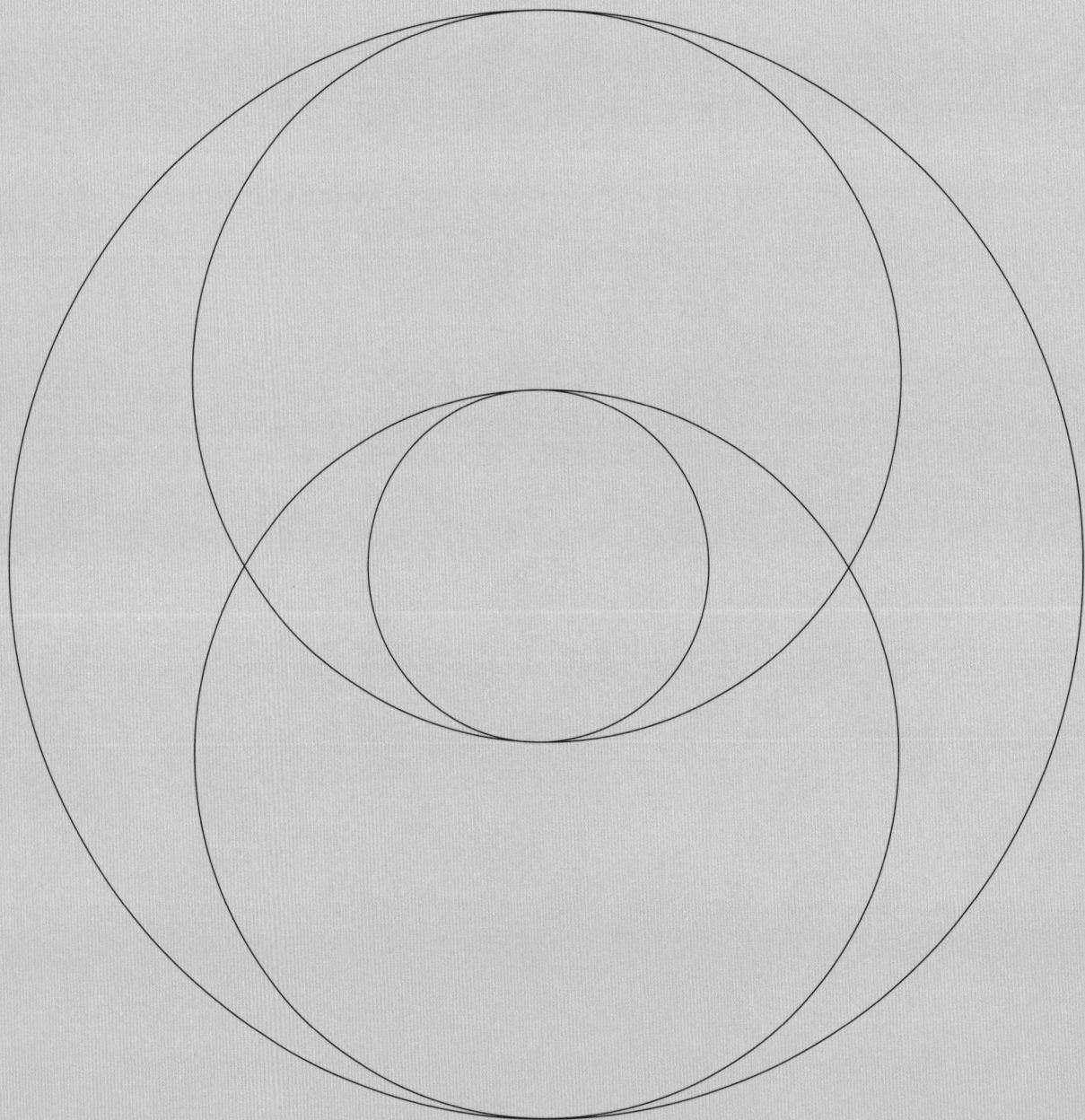

If we allow it to, nature can teach us many things. Some would say everything that we need answers to can be found in nature as it is the origin of many of life's essentials, such as nutrition, medicine and materials.

The wisdom that I use every day in my work has been passed down for generations through medicine women, shamans and healers. How did they find the solutions to so many ailments without the use of chemistry, biology and physics? It is simple: by observing and being a part of nature, the answers eventually come.

We can also learn deeply about ourselves from nature by observing animals, plants, seasons and the sky. Seeing these rhythms and the pace of the natural world can be an anchor for us. Catastrophes can strike and yet, nature keeps on going. Every day the Sun will rise and fall no matter what unfolded the day before.

Over the years I have looked forward to watching birds and whales migrating, signaling the change of season. When the sky turns a particular shade of greeny grey I know it will hail, and when the hairs on my arms stand on end I know lightning is close by. I've learnt to smell the rain coming.

Nature can impart wisdom to anyone who listens. But to listen, that is the true wisdom.

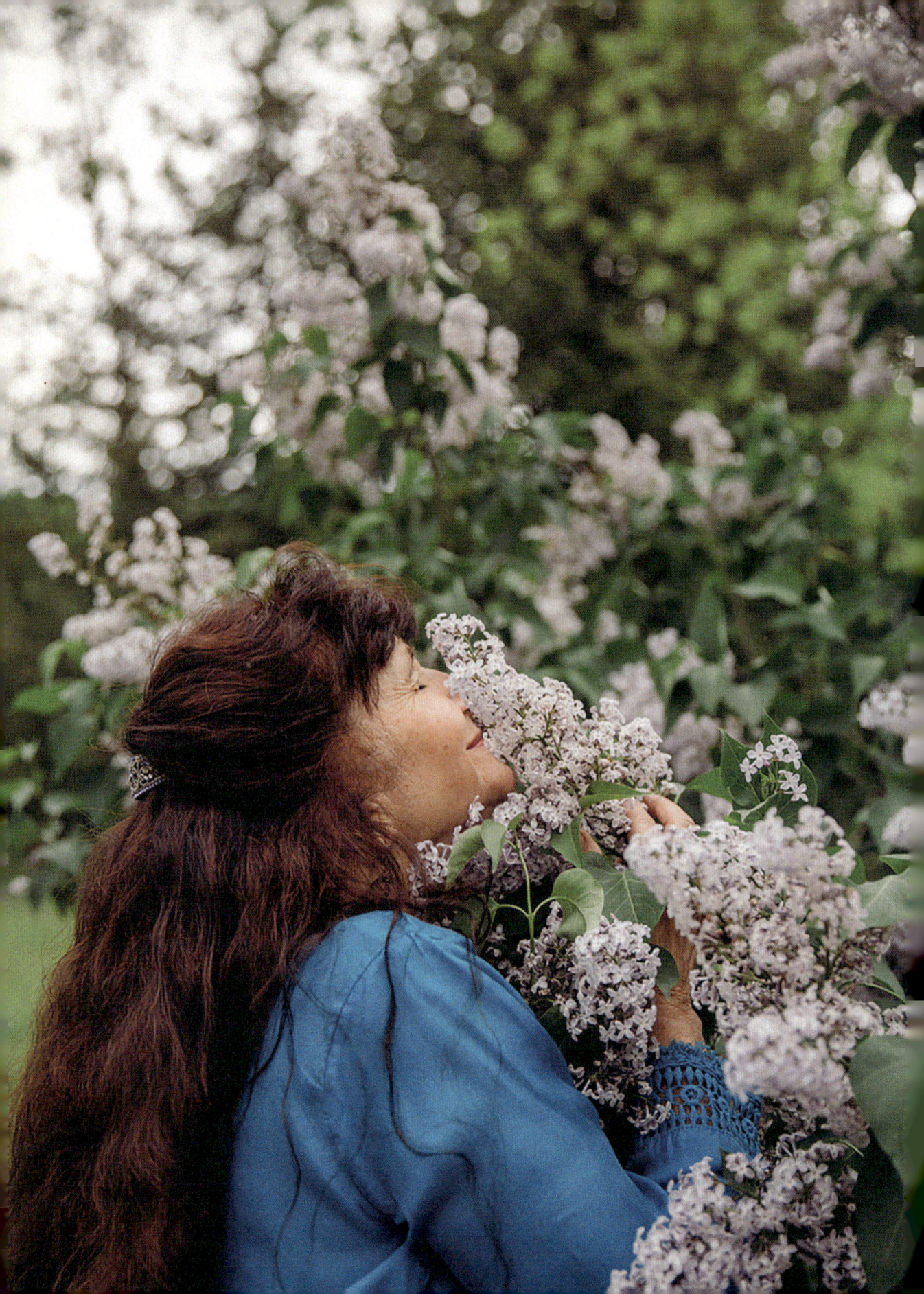

Herbalism

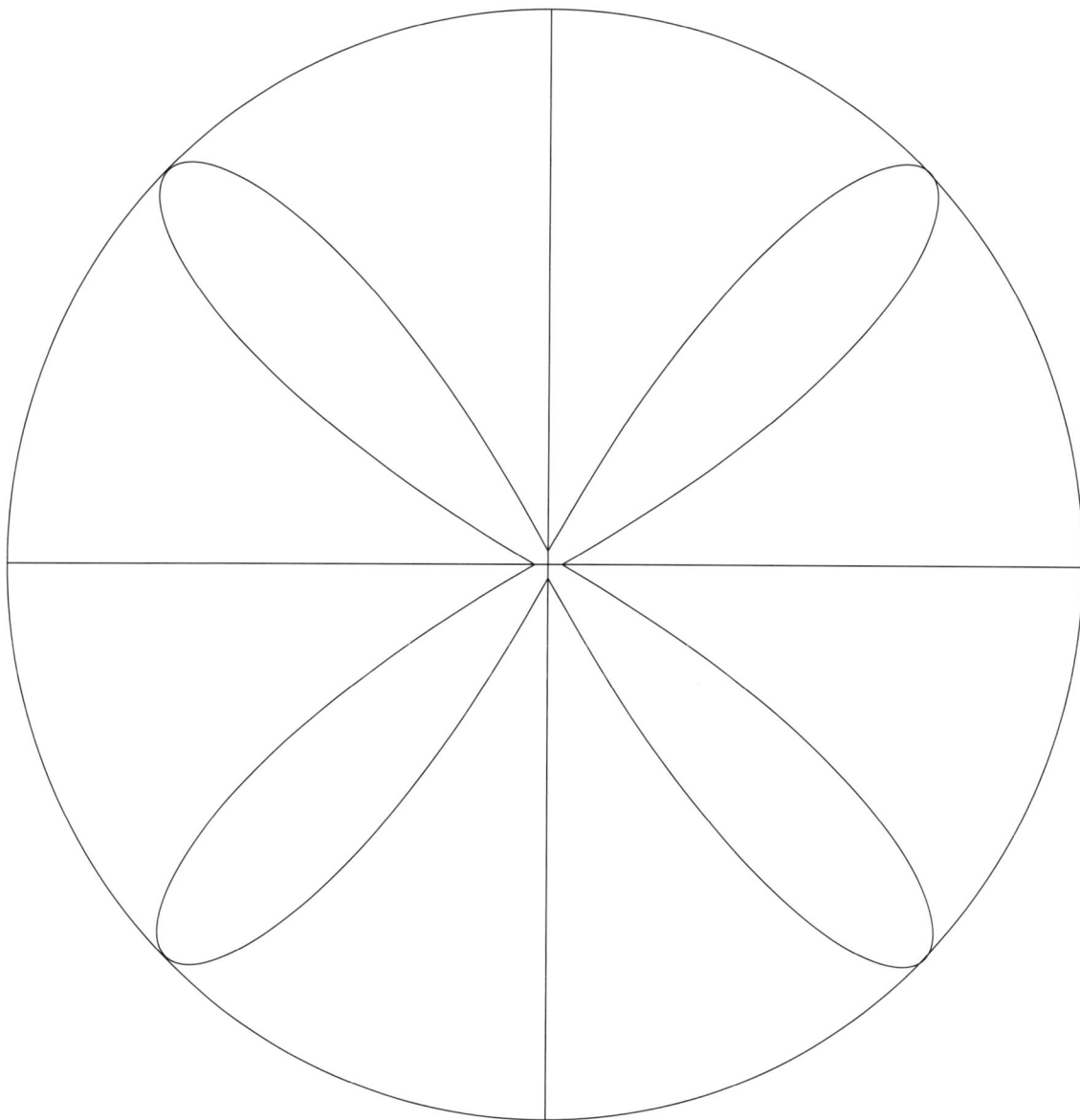

Harnessing herbal medicine to ignite inner wisdom

Rosemary Gladstar

● USA

'There is a much greater sense of harmony and diversity between plants than we see among people. You look at any garden, whether it's cultivated or wild, it thrives better in diversity: nature knows that … nature does better.'

It seems that everywhere Rosemary Gladstar has been, a trail of plants and beauty is left in her wake. Her first herb shop, first herb school and even the dairy farm she grew up on as a child (which is now a plant nursery) are all still flourishing. In her eighth decade on this Earth, Rosemary humbly reflects on the strong legacy she has built within the world of herbal medicine and nature connection. While she is most known for the many books she has written and the education programs she facilitates, Rosemary considers herself a lover of nature.

'Some people have called me an entrepreneur because I've been successful with herbal businesses. That's all okay with me, but I think of myself as a simple Earth person who loves plants. I'm a plant lover even more than the term herbalist.'

Rosemary grew up in Northern California, USA, on a farm called Wildwood Dairy. She remembers running through the fields with her brothers and sisters and climbing into a big willow tree where she would stay until after dark. 'I was kind of afraid of the cows. I remember being up in the tree and feeling utter safety. I can still close my eyes and remember that sensation: knowing that tree was alive and protecting me, never wanting to come out of that tree. Those are my earliest memories of being protected and held and feeling safe,' she says, recounting where her initial love of nature unfolded.

While her enjoyment for the outdoors grew organically, Rosemary credits her grandmother with sparking her interest in using plants for medicine. Fleeing from the Armenian genocide to the United States, Rosemary's grandmother always said that along with her faith, her knowledge of plants is what kept her alive. This sentiment of knowing how to gather your own food and medicine was passed down to her grandchildren, but it was Rosemary who took the keenest interest. 'We'd be outside helping her garden. She'd pull the weeds out and put them into the food basket, telling us how she would cook them and use them. It stuck with me, even when I was really little. It became part of who I was.'

As a young girl, Rosemary was already set on her path, featuring her local plants in as many of her school reports as she could. Upon finishing high school she knew that herbal medicine was the only path for her. In 1972 her first shop, Rosemary's Garden, now considered a herbalist mecca in California, was opened. It didn't take long for Rosemary to begin teaching her community about the plants she was offering and how they too could use herbal medicine. 'People were really craving this information; they were missing the connection with Earth. I never imagined myself teaching, even to this day, having to get up in front of people and talk, I have to take lots of kava (a herb to calm the nervous system) and I'm always really nervous.'

What started out as eight people in her house with her grandmother cooking wild herb stew for everyone, eventually prospered into a herb school, a distance education program, twice yearly herbal conferences and countless seminars and lectures. Rosemary's approach is traditional, intuitive and tactile, something that she believes is essential for the modern herbalist. 'It is important for

The wisdom of nature

people to get out into the garden and actually listen to the plants. I really value all the research and scientific studies that are coming up, I think it's fabulous as long as it augments wisdom.'

Her ethos is simply to spark ancestral knowledge within her students. 'There are lots of different ways we do that because everybody is so different. Some might be at a herb walk, others might be sitting and meditating with the plants; some are working hands-on with the plants and others are engaged thinking about the chemical constituents, and then all of a sudden, spark spark spark.'

In 1987 Rosemary pivoted and left California for the forests of Vermont at Sage Mountain Botanical Sanctuary, a rugged wilderness retreat for herbalists. 'It was a wonderful experience to come to that mountain, people thought they were signing up to take courses with me but really that was just a front, they were really coming to study with the mountain. The mountain was the sage,' she says. However, after over three decades spent on Sage Mountain, Rosemary and her husband have recently passed on the stewardship of the land to live a simpler life by Lake Champlain. 'When I was full-time teaching, travelling and writing, I found myself starting to lose my connection. It was a physical thing for me, I couldn't hear the plants talking in my head anymore ... I'm grateful that I was able to do it but I'm also grateful that I knew when it was time to stop.'

Rosemary notes that she has now come full circle and gone back to what she was doing fifty years ago – growing herbs and making things for her community. 'What is so interesting is that herbal medicine started from the ground up rather than from the medical society. It had a much more earthy way of presenting itself – it was more about people's medicine. You could grow this medicine, you could wildcraft it, you could make it for nothing. If you were poor, you had medicine. It became much more doable for the regular person.'

She would never admit it, but Rosemary is a big reason why herbalism in the USA is such a robust and continually growing craft. While there was certainly a movement in the 1960s and 1970s for earth-based practices, without her dedication to guiding the everyday person, this wisdom may have been lost.

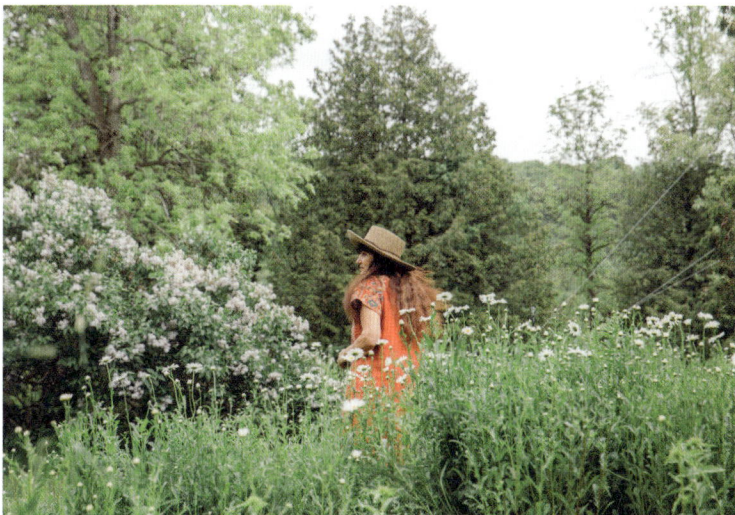

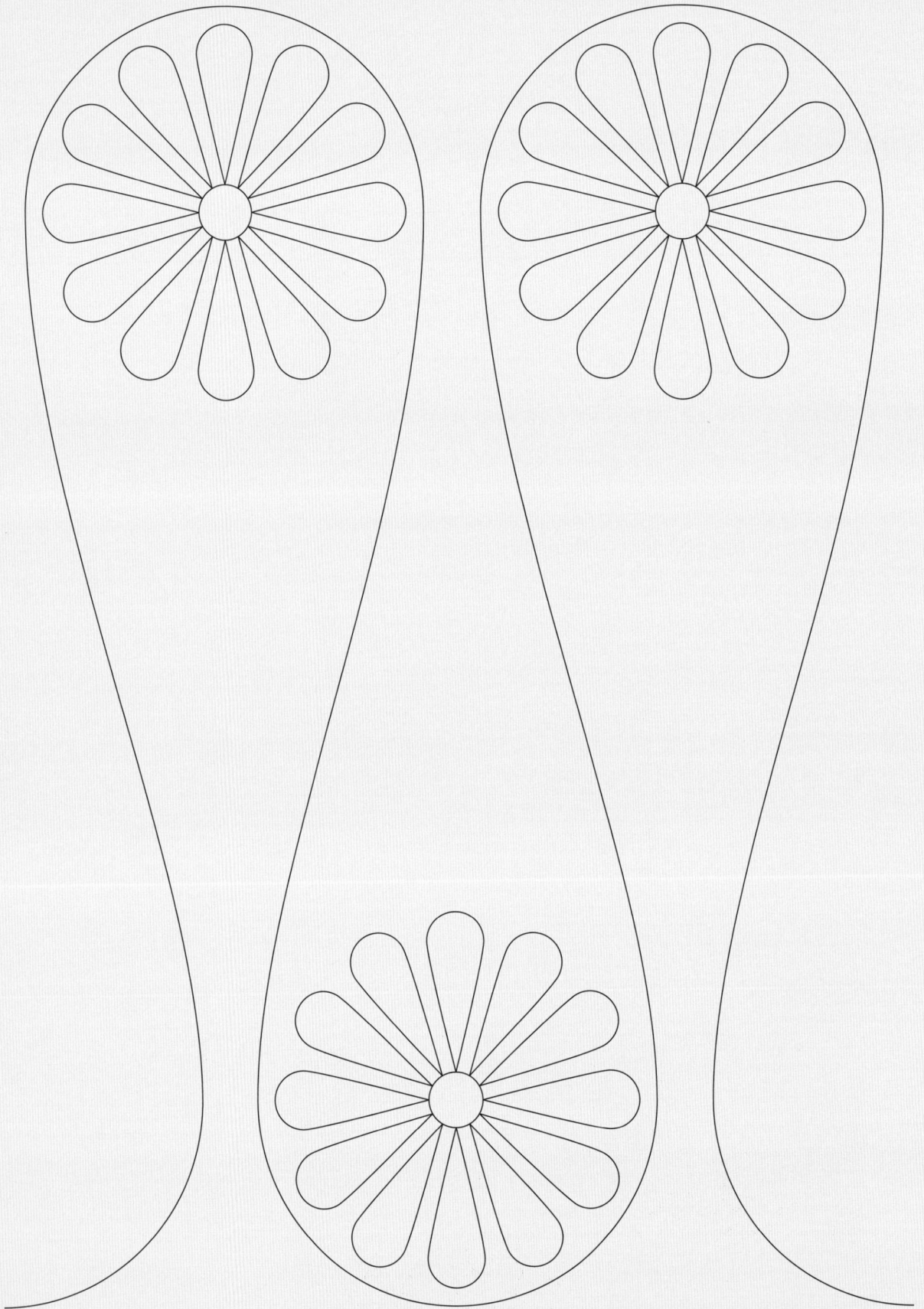

Plant meditation for feeling grounded and expansive

Inspired by Rosemary Gladstar

Meditation is a practice that has been part of human history for thousands of years in different expressions. They may not have called it such but many of our ancient cultures had some form of meditative or mindfulness-based tradition. What was once considered a spiritual or religious practice in our modern history has now transformed into a lifestyle tool that can benefit both physical and mental health.

Research into meditation has shown that it can:

- reduce anxiety
- improve mental clarity
- better your sleep quality
- decrease stress levels
- boost self-worth
- lower blood pressure
- minimise levels of pain
- enhance your immune system's activity.

Meditation is a technique that can be taught to anyone and there are no barriers to try it. You don't need a fancy cushion, prayer beads or an experienced teacher to meditate. Although, if you want those, go right ahead.

There are many types of meditation available to explore and experiment with, such as counting your breath, reciting a mantra (sacred word or phrase) and walking meditation. The one thing all of these practices have in common is the goal to bring the meditator back into the present moment. Rather than eliminating all thoughts, the purpose is to recognise when you are lost in the endless stream of thoughts. Recognising your internal dialogue and having just a small glimmer of presence is what even the most experienced meditators are working towards.

$\longrightarrow$

To begin ●

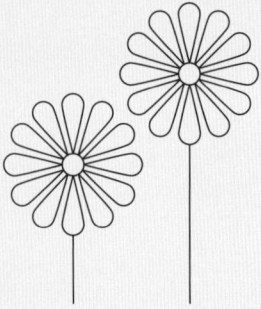

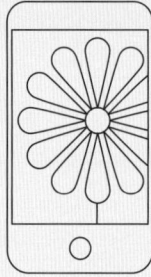

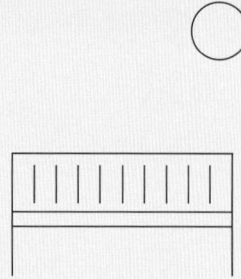

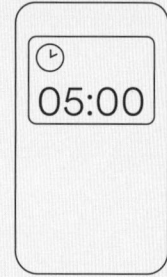

● 1
Choose a plant that you feel drawn to. It could be a flower you see on your daily walk, a herb you use in cooking or a succulent growing in your home.

● 2
If the plant is moveable, or you can take a fallen leaf or flower, that would work well. Otherwise, take a photograph of the plant and bring it with you.

● 3
Find a place where you can sit for your meditation with minimal disturbances. This can be done anywhere but doing it outside can really enhance the experience.

● 4
Sit or lay in a position that is comfortable for you to maintain for at least five minutes.

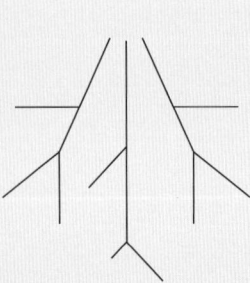

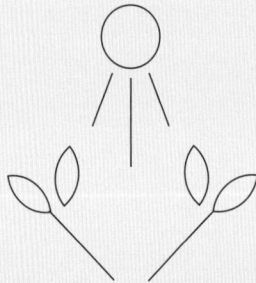

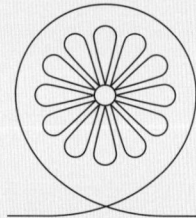

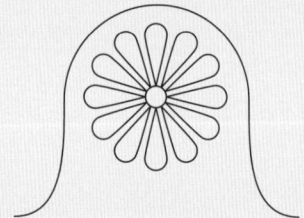

● 9
Imagine you have roots growing out of the bottom of your body deep into the soil. The roots slowly continue moving down, giving you stability and strength.

● 10
Imagine your limbs are branches and leaves absorbing sunlight to help you grow. They are curious, courageous and expansive.

● 11
As you breathe in, you are connecting with the core of the plant and its purpose.

● 12
As you breathe out, you are connecting with the outward expression of the plant and its beauty.

The wisdom of nature

5

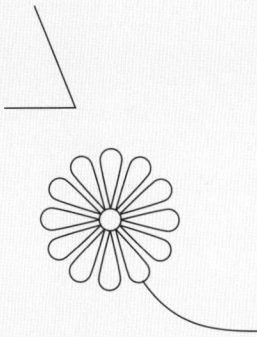

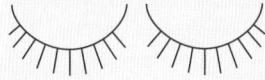

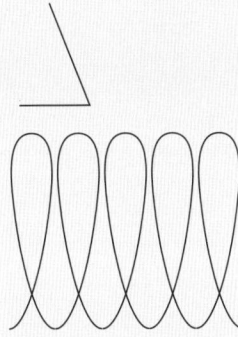

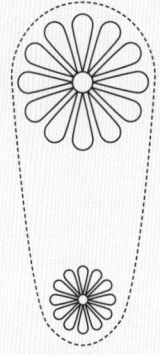

Spend a few minutes connecting with your plant. If it's with you, touch its leaves or petals, smell it, breathe it in. If you only have your photograph, really observe all of the colours and textures you can see.

6

Now close your eyes and allow your body to become still and relaxed.

7

Take five deep belly breaths in and out of your nose.

8

Picture yourself as the plant you are connecting with, expanding both upwards towards the sky and down into the depths of Earth.

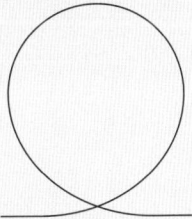

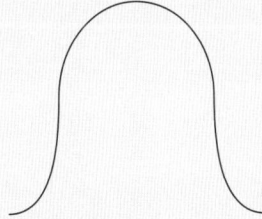

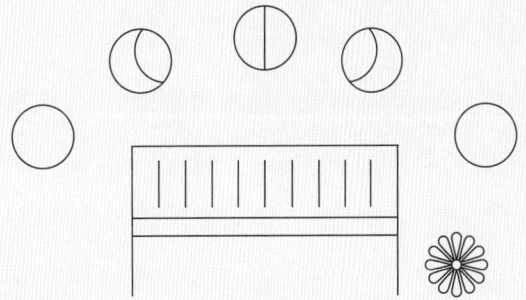

13

Breathe in and feel grounded in your place.

14

Breathe out and feel that you are expanding and flourishing.

15

Continue this meditation for as long as you like.

16

Try to repeat this process consecutively for a number of days or weeks with the same plant and notice how your relationship to it changes over time. How would it feel to be this connected to all plants?

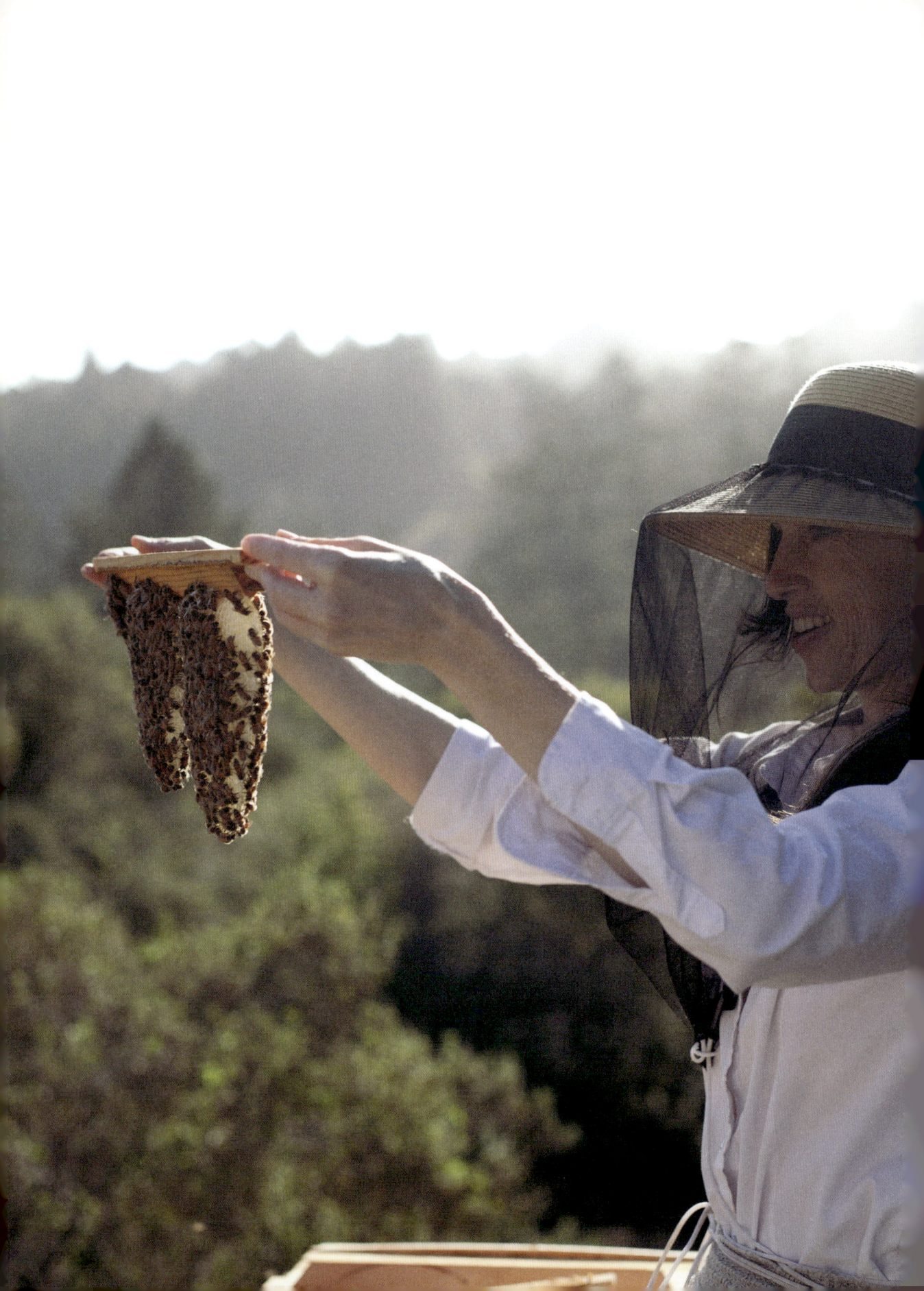

Beekeeping

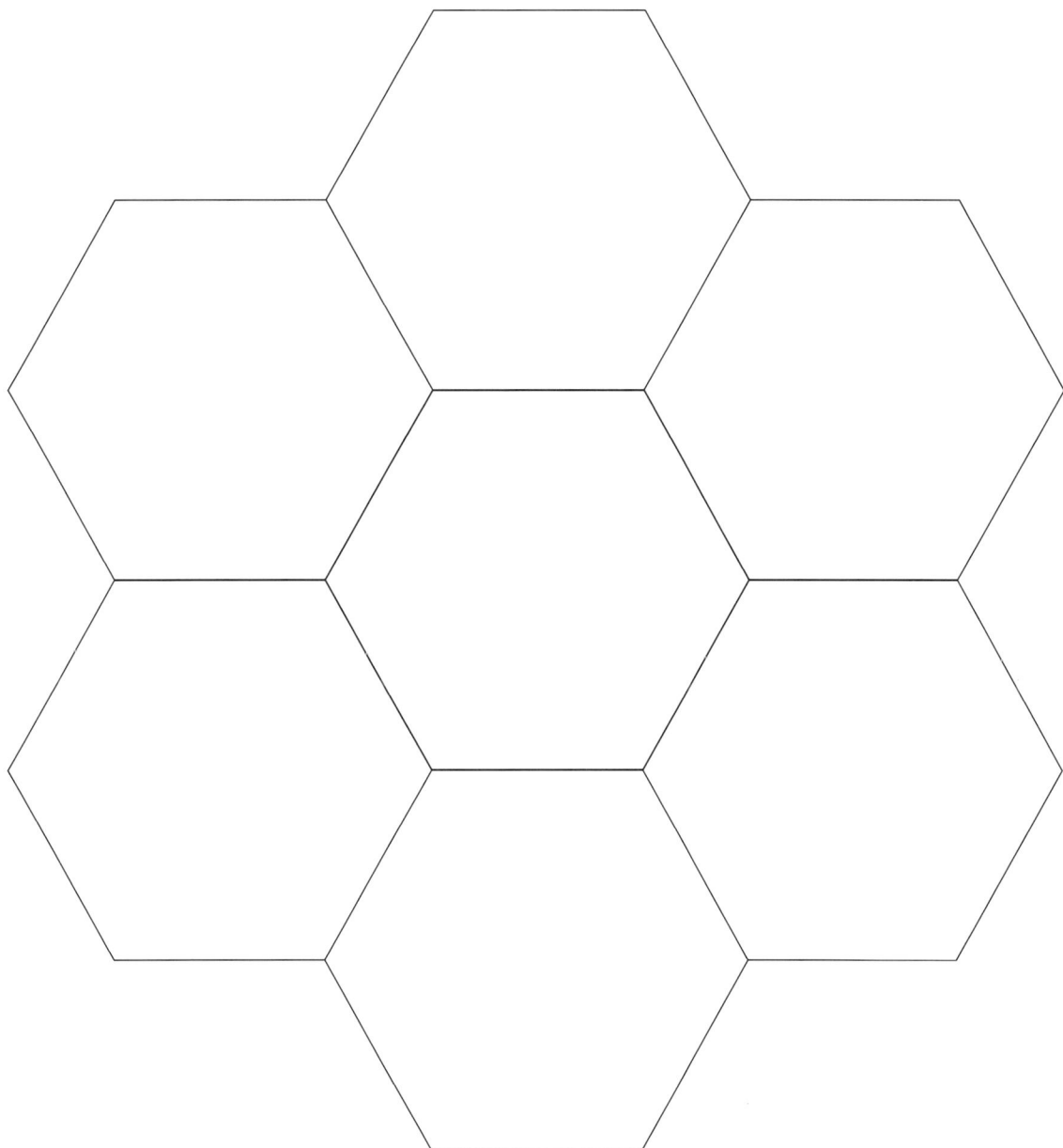

Caring for bees as a form of mindfulness

Ariella Daly

● UK

'If you're paying attention you don't need to get stung because the bees are going to tap you near your head or your gloves to let you know you're not fully on board right now, come back.'

As an anthropology student exploring folkloric traditions of Europe, Ariella Daly came across an ancient practice that involved beekeeping. She took part in a workshop in the United Kingdom to learn what she thought would be predominantly intellectual facts. Instead, she became fascinated with the lineages of women who tended to bees since as far back as ancient Greek times. 'I went, not with a connection to bees but with a tug that I want to understand this folk tradition. While I was there, a swarm of bees moved into a wall of my house, behind my bedroom.'

Thus began Ariella's relationship with bees. 'It was synchronistic, but it wasn't intentional,' she says. During that same year and in swarm season as well, Ariella miscarried after three months. 'It's a very specific window of time in the spring. I remember praying and beseeching whatever was out there to bring me something I could mother, and bees showed up in an apple tree a week later.' This time in Ariella's life was full of grief and deep healing, but it was the bees that helped remedy her pain.

It was this healing potential that originally helped foster Ariella's initial interest in bees. 'The thing about bees is that they require a kind of presence that doesn't allow you to be checked out of your body.' Ariella was feeling disassociated from her body but because of the presence required for tending her bees, she found her way back to herself. 'The bees will let you know if you're not present through a wonderful mechanism known as the sting.'

After everything she had experienced, Ariella was forced to make a decision: to pursue the path of beekeeping or to continue what she had been doing. 'I was a performing artist but there was a fork in the road where it was either music or bees. I chose bees because they brought me back to life when I was suffering so greatly.'

Ariella now practises natural beekeeping or bee-centric beekeeping which focuses more on the health of the bees and building natural habitats rather than honey cultivation or pollination for monocrops. This practice has developed because of the importance of bees to our own survival. 'Without bees we will be severely affected as the bees pollinate Earth and pollination creates our food,' she says. 'The way that we have been farming is out of balance and the bees are suffering as a result. There are a lot more diseases spreading and weakened genetics that the bees are losing the traits that help them survive.'

She highlights how the treatment of bees reflects how we also look at other areas of life. 'There are so many parallels with beekeeping and health, beekeeping and the feminine and women's bodies, and even in how we parent,' says Ariella. For us to do better in these areas a different kind of approach is required. 'There are many pathways of knowing and learning: things like meditation, intuition, the sense of feeling, and the body as an informant.' By strengthening these skills, we can live more aligned with how the bees experience the world – living in harmony with their environment.

Keeping bees can be a way of enhancing these deeper ways of knowing. Interacting with bees means interacting with the whole hive as they function as one super-organism. 'Collectively as an organism, they are aware and give information to the rest of the hive about what's going on in their environment, including when a human comes near their hive,' she says. 'They read the heat signature of your face and body, your body movements and how you're breathing. They are very sensitive to how you're interacting and there's a tonal shift in the way the bees sound. When the bees are in a happy humming state, it's one of the most calming sounds to the human nervous system.'

Ariella talks fondly of new therapies being developed in Europe which use the hum of bees to aid mental health – done by placing hives underneath bedrooms in treatment centres. While this may not be widely available yet, Ariella says that any one of us can keep bees. 'I have found that some of the most prolific, healthiest hives are on rooftops in cities because people garden in the cities,' she says. 'The biggest issue is if there are enough flowers, so if you're not sure, plant flowers.'

From having a fear of nature, due to a traumatic experience with a snake as a child, to now interacting daily with creatures many of us keep at arm's length, Ariella is a testament to how potent the scary bits of nature can be. 'Things that were insurmountable in the past became attainable. It's not so much because of bees but it's as if they became an anchor for me in my life and a lens through which I could see abundance and beauty.' A large part of that beauty was the birth of her child, ten years on from having her miscarriage and becoming a beekeeper.

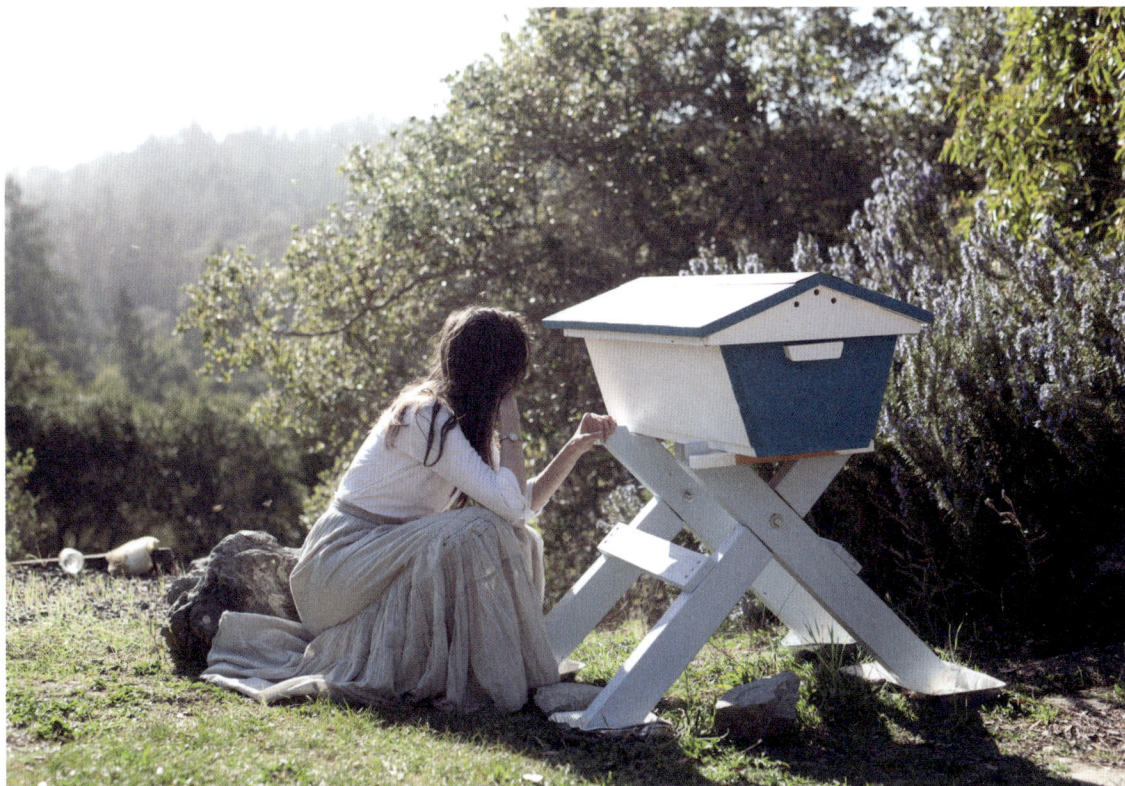

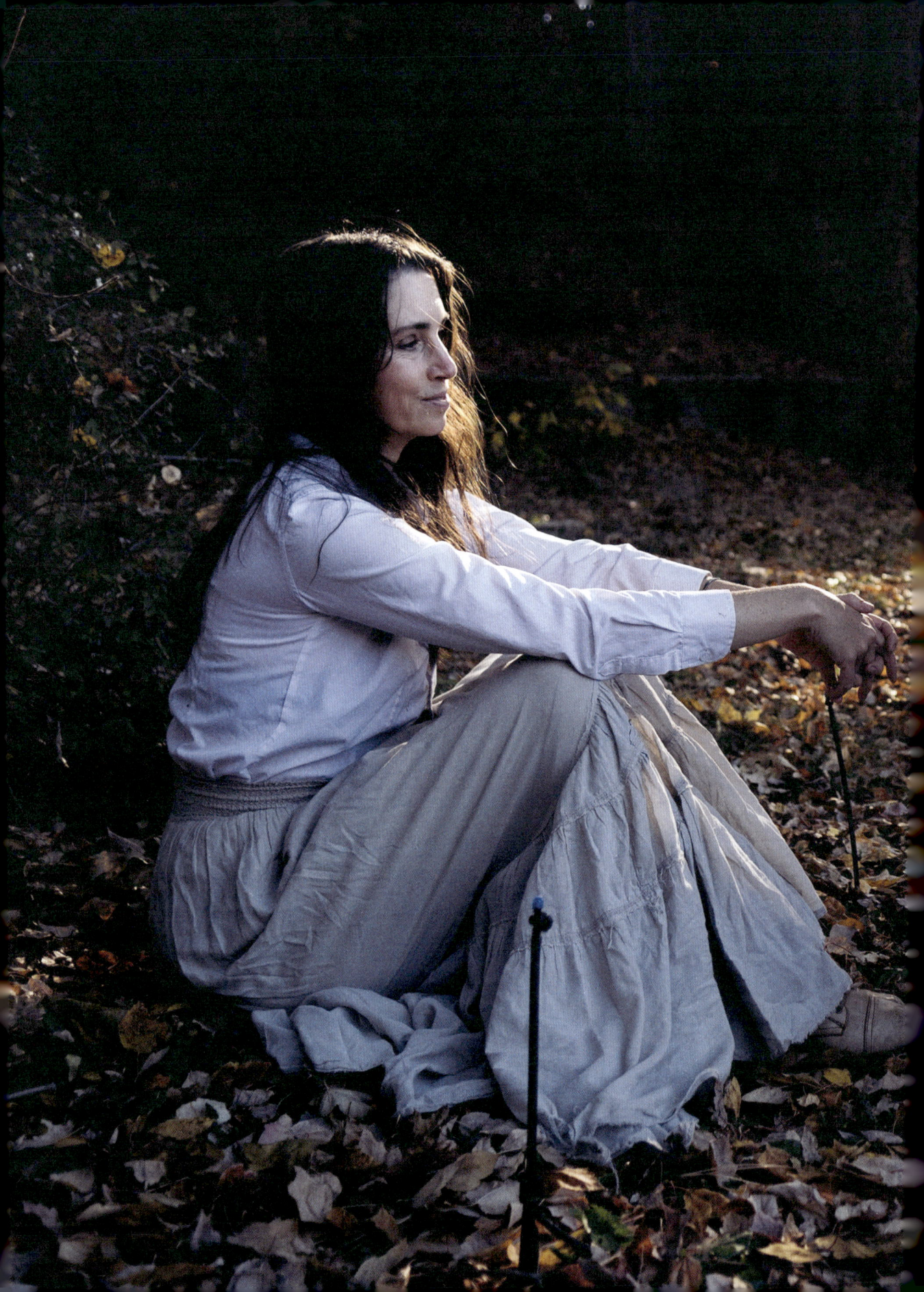

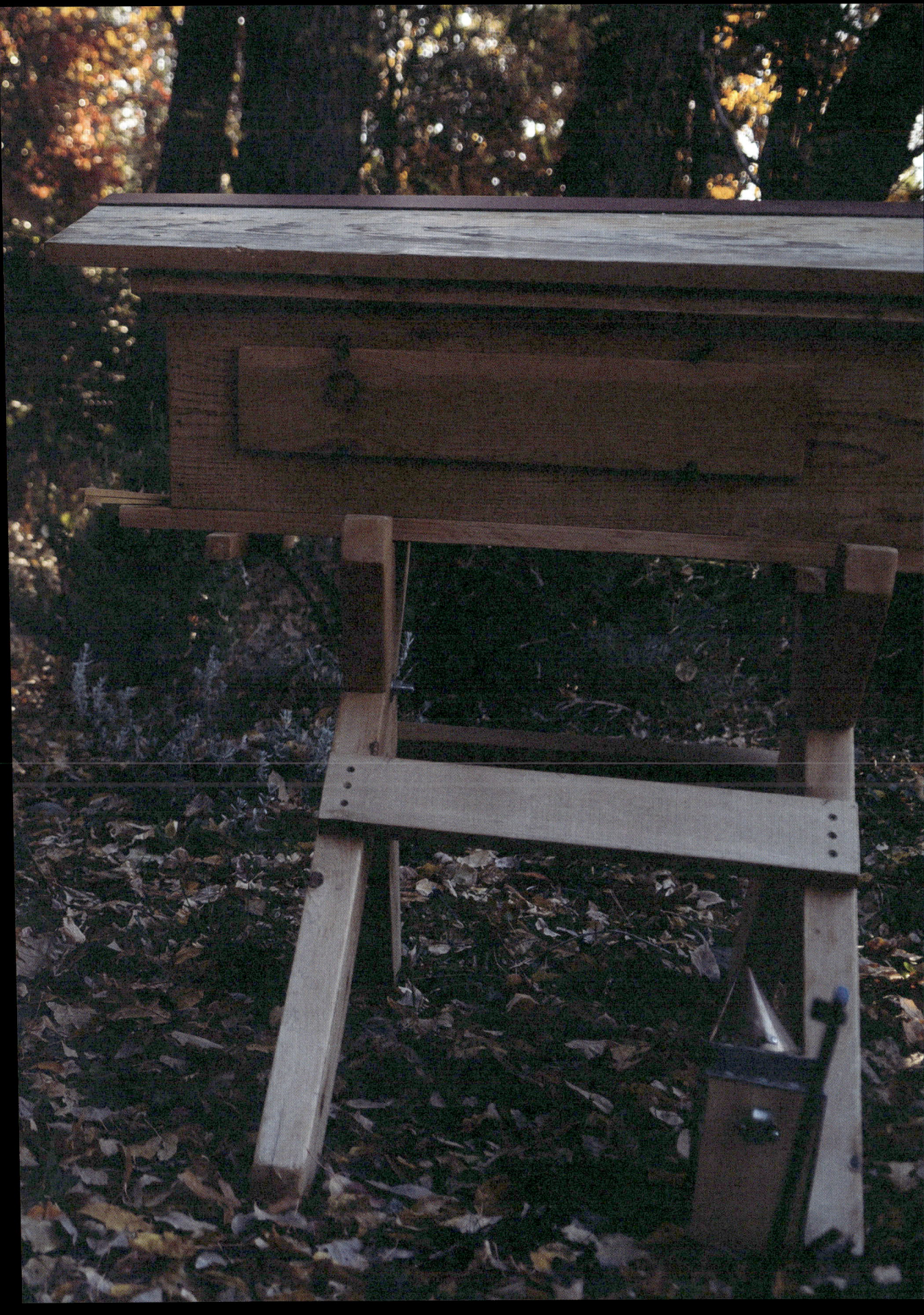

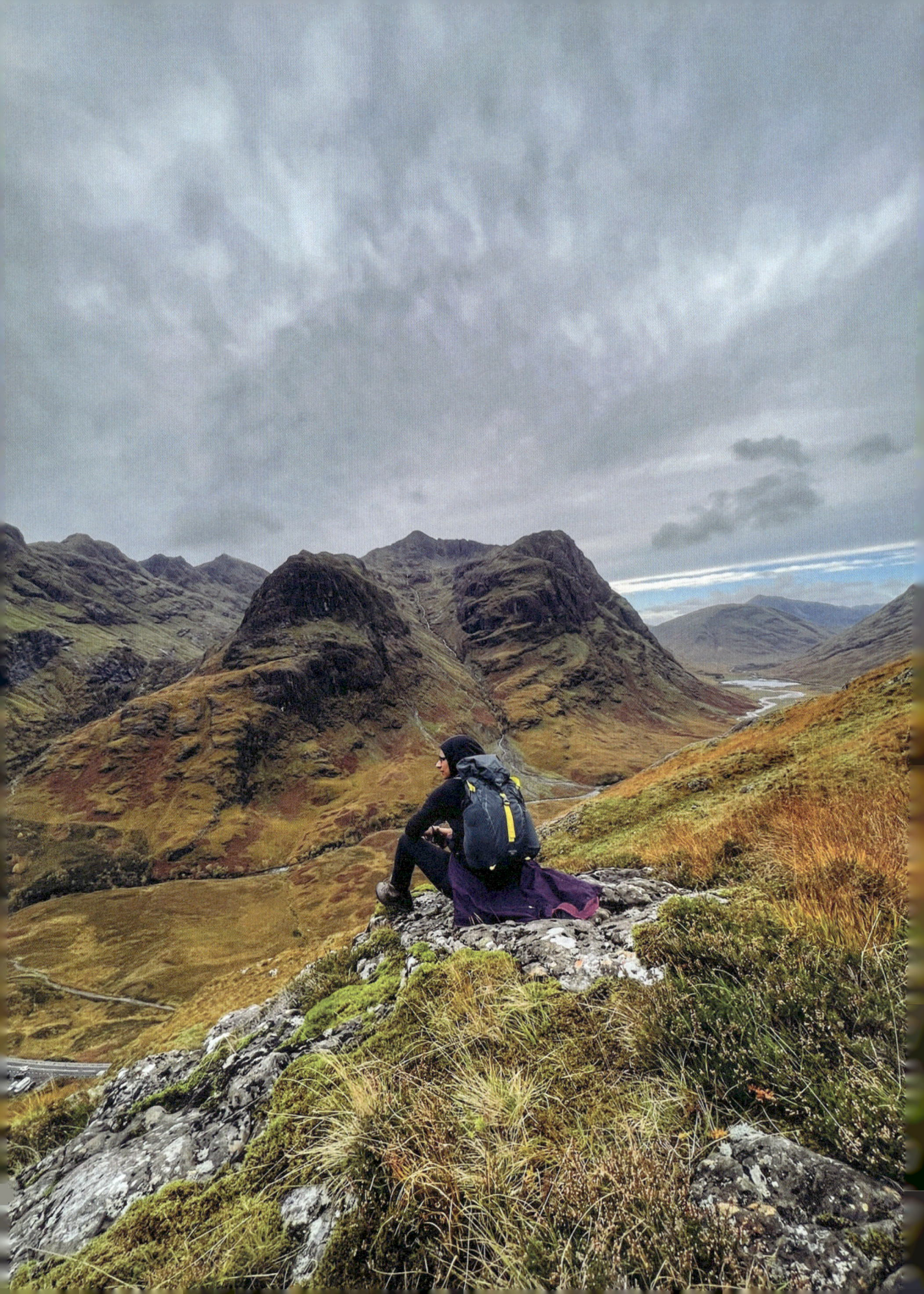

Group adventures

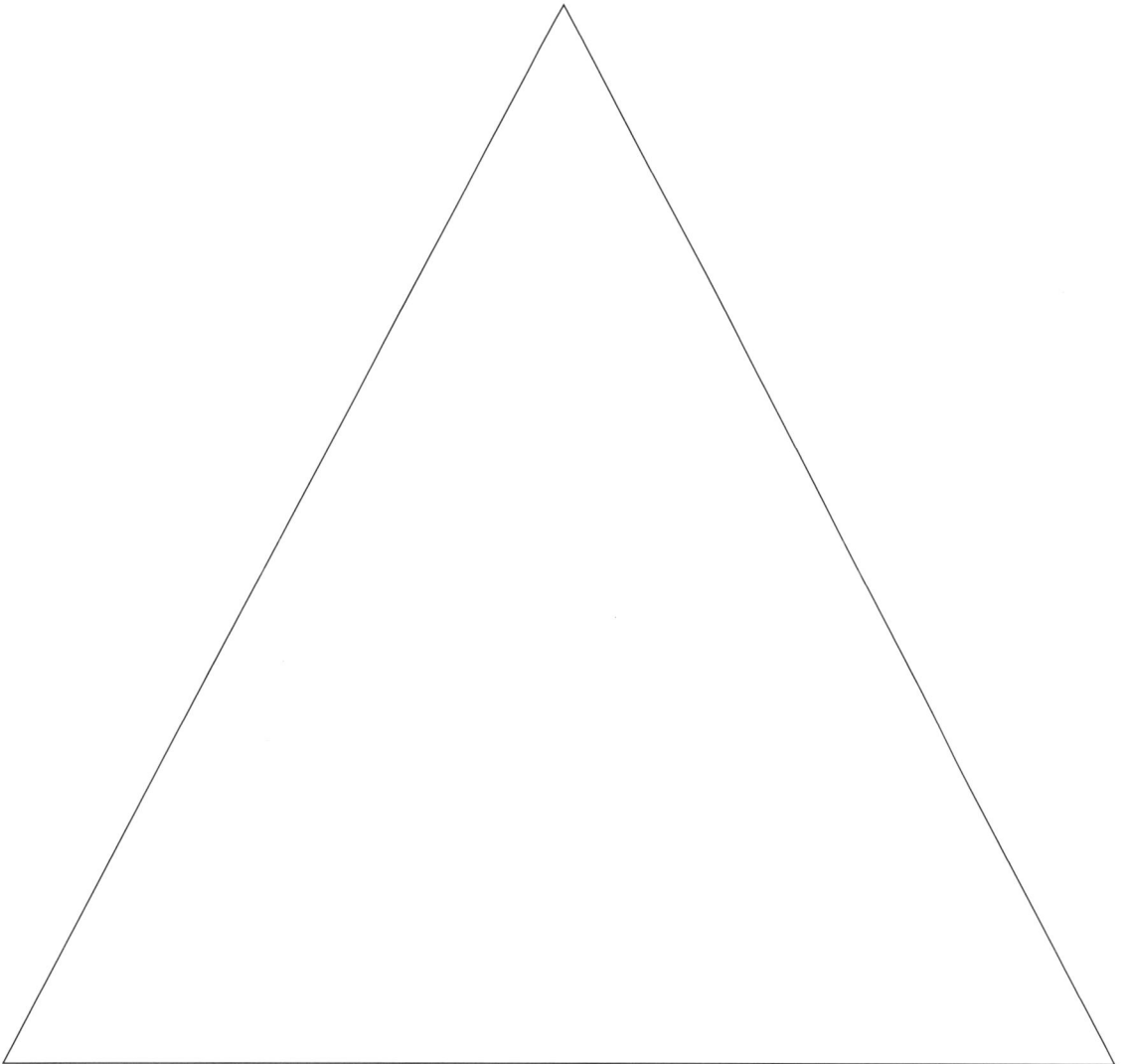

Guided hiking for generational change and strengthening faith

Aysha Sharif

● UK

Unlike other members in her hiking group for Muslim women, Aysha Sharif grew up in an 'outdoorsy' family. Her dad, as a teenager, came to the United Kingdom from a farming community in Pakistan and was used to spending time outdoors on his own. Aysha cherishes the memories of her and her family camping and hiking a couple of times a year, but hiking with people outside of the family unit was not encouraged by her community. As an adult, Aysha experienced a great deal of cultural backlash when she first started solo hiking as a divorced woman and single mum. 'I never want my daughters to feel that. I battled it out and I really pushed so that they could have a better life. That's what these adventures tied into: it was a push against culture.'

Hearing the things people in her community would say about her caused Aysha a great deal of anxiety and mental suffering. 'I remember the first few times I went solo hiking. I used to hide my boots and then get changed in the car,' she says, 'but then I thought I'm not doing anything wrong. I'm not doing anything that goes against my religion so why do I feel so guilty? It's because I was resisting everything that culture said.' Finding the strength to carry on was for the benefit of her daughters and other women in her community, a sentiment that has carried forward into the ethos of her hiking group, The Wanderlust Women.

Aysha first met Amira Patel, the founder of The Wanderlust Women, when she moved to the Lakes District of Northern England in 2020. Initially the group was set up as a way for Amira to meet other Muslim women and experience the outdoors together, but it has now grown to mean so much more. 'These women, they start getting empowered. And for us it's not just hiking, it's not just taking a woman up a mountain, it's about empowering that woman.' Aysha has witnessed the potent knock-on effects of that empowerment many times over. 'For us, it's more than the woman who attends the event, it's what she goes home and teaches her daughters, her family and her community. It's how she empowers them too.'

'Sometimes it's just showing people that they can do more, that they aren't restricted by their own thoughts. When you are surrounded by people who think like you, the same thought patterns keep getting recycled again and again. That's why it's so important that these groups keep happening, because it brings fresh ideas to women.'

The Wanderlust Women have been successful in adapting to the logistical hurdles of praying on a mountain or in the outdoors. 'A lot of women struggle with the connection between faith and the outdoors. We pray five times a day and if you're on a mountain for six or seven hours, most likely you are going to experience at least two of the prayers up there. You can go canyoning and rock climbing and you don't have to turn your back on your faith.' To aid this The Wanderlust Women created portable prayer kits with prayer mats that are waterproof, a mini hijab which can be put over existing clothes, and ablution equipment. They are also collaborating with hiking brands to make more modest clothing options for all different body types so the women in their groups can feel comfortable going on expeditions.

The wisdom of nature

Knowing that they don't have to choose between conserving their modesty or wearing heavy undesirable clothing is part of breaking down the barrier for Muslim women to enjoy the outdoors.

While they may have overcome many obstacles, Aysha says there is still the unfamiliarity of seeing Muslim women on a trail, especially in the United Kingdom, that can feel uncomfortable. She recalls a time when solo hiking in Wales and a man on the trail stopped her, questioning her ability to get to the top of the mountain. 'I made it my mission to beat him. Even though I was tired and wanted to take my time, I had to get there before him. And I did. It's little microaggressions like that that make you feel like you have to prove you are deserving of this space.'

Nature has been a huge support for Aysha during times of self-worry or doubt. She compares the way nature grows as a source of inspiration for how we can live our lives and she tries to impart this wisdom to her hiking groups. 'A tree has grown without anybody's permission and its branches have curved in a way that didn't need anybody's input. If you allow yourself to flow through life the way water flows then you don't get cortisol (stress hormone) spikes. You don't get the migraines or the anxiety because you're not forcing things; you're allowing things just like nature intended.'

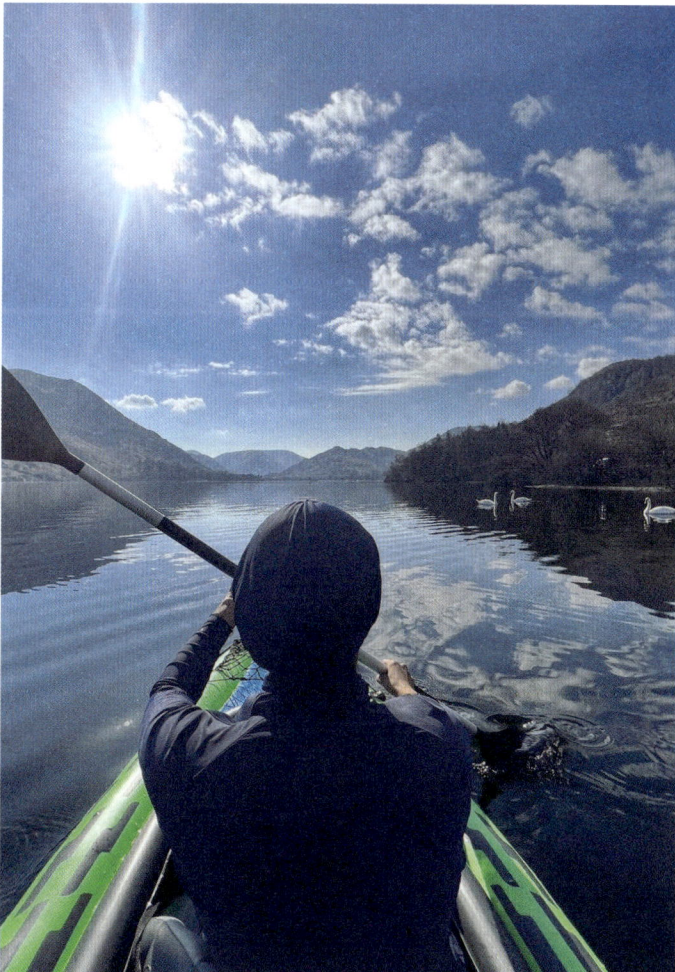

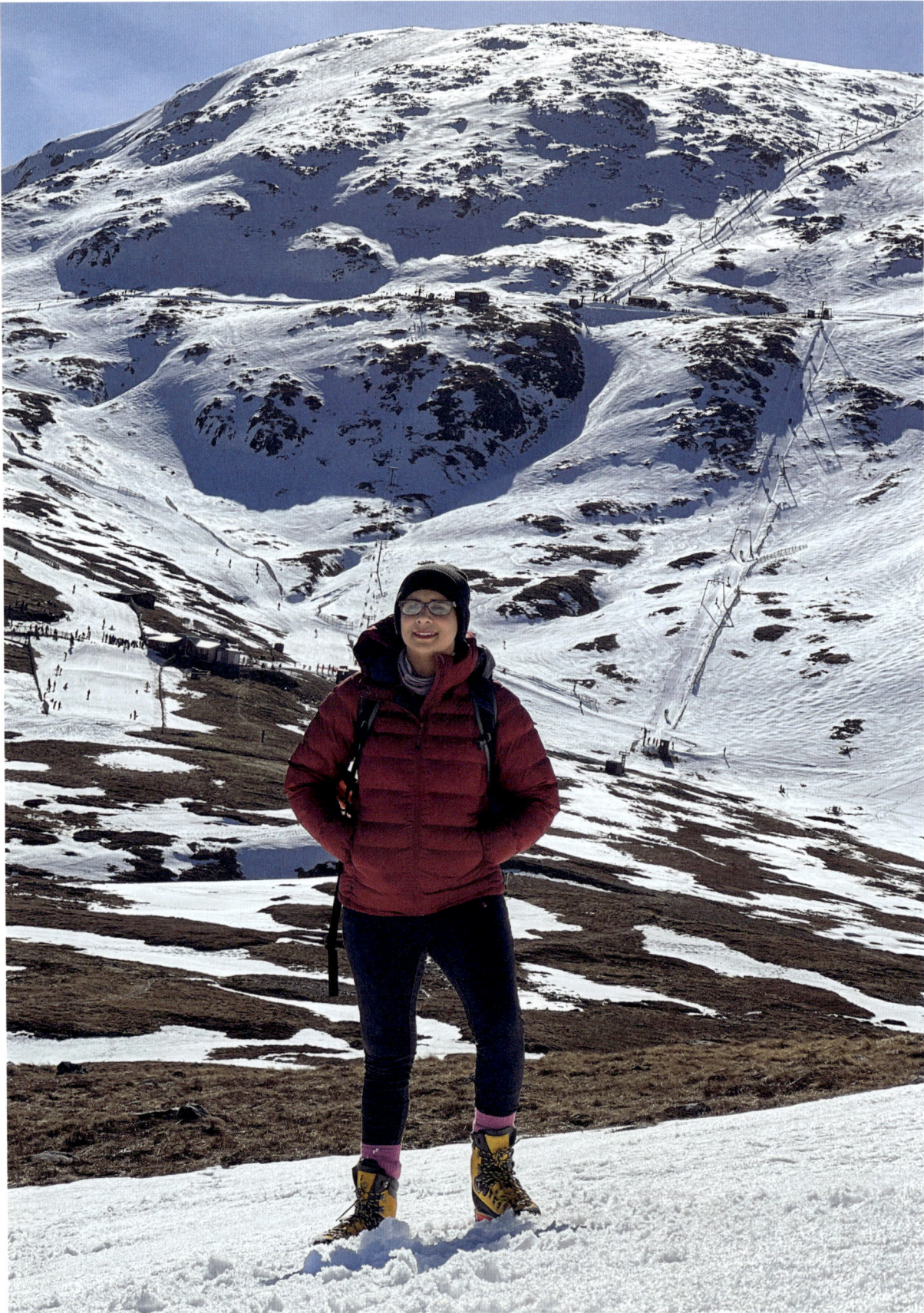

'When you go up a mountain
with a problem, you come
down with a solution.'

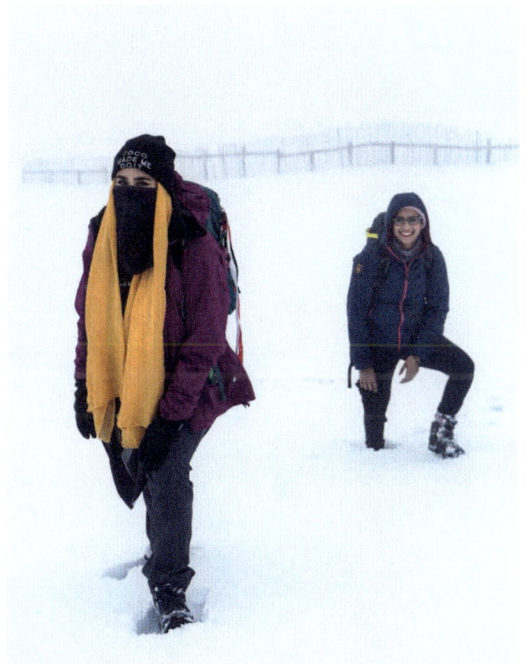

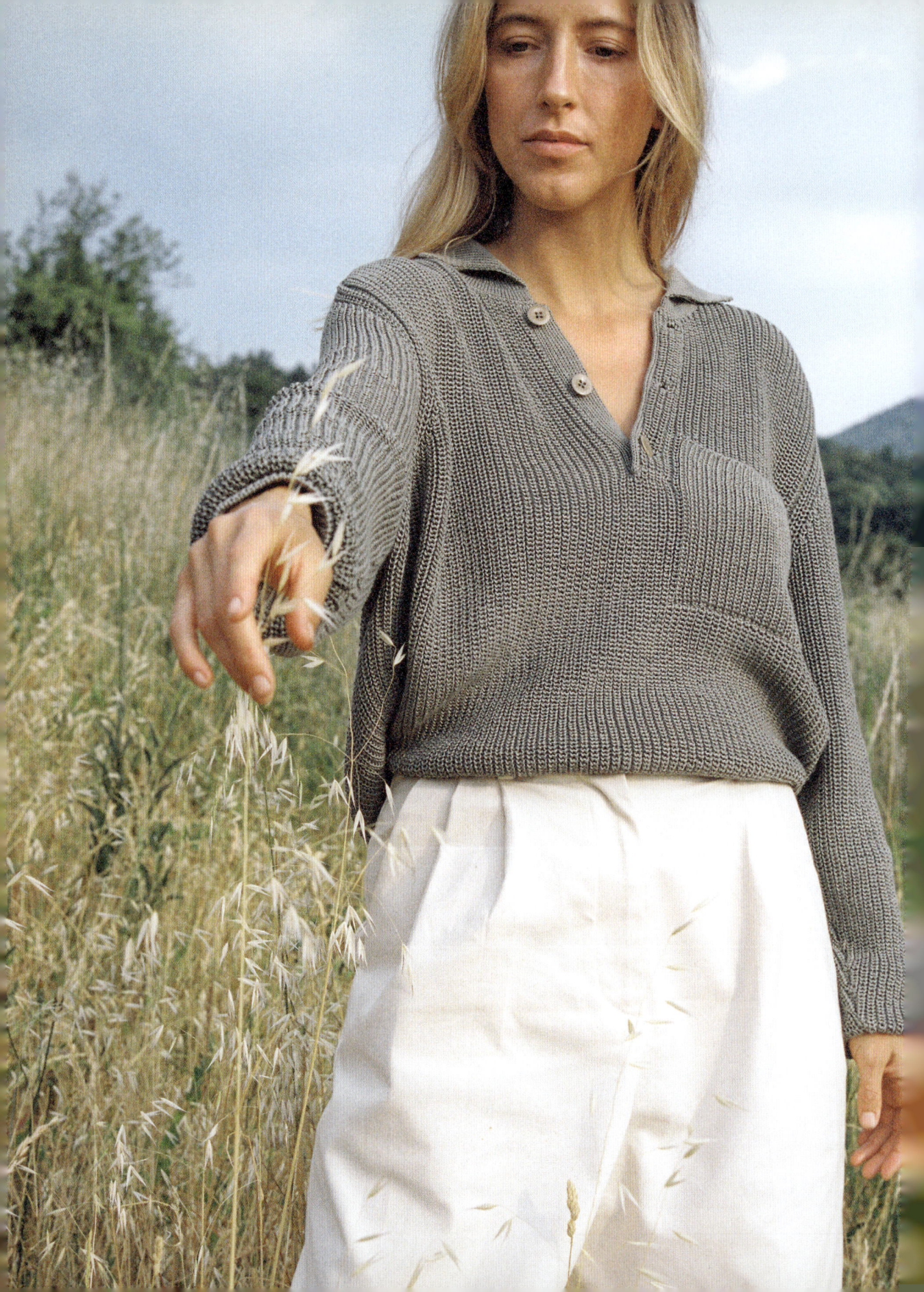

Self-sufficient living

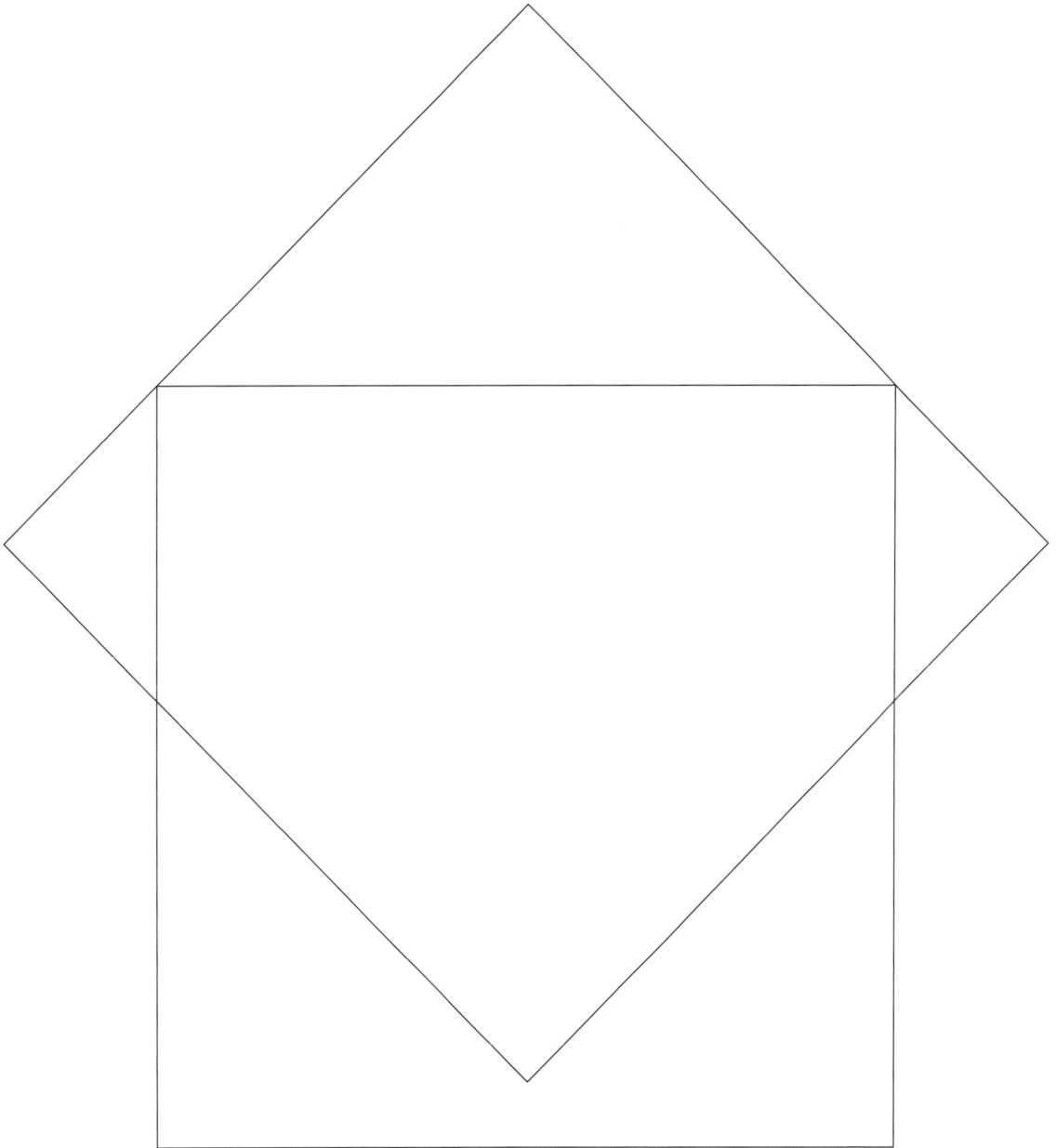

Following rewilding practices to cultivate freedom

Anya Lily Montague

● Italy

What was meant to be a trip of only a few weeks to visit some land her brother purchased in Tuscany, Italy, turned into a complete reshape of Anya Lily Montague's life. She was blown away when she arrived and quickly realised she wasn't going to leave, and she hasn't since. 'There was so much potential for healing and learning,' she says, 'I asked my brother if I could start a retreat here and he said "of course, my place is your place".' This is how Meadowsweet Retreat, a rewilding live-in experience for guests was born.

Prior to coming to Tuscany, Anya had been feeling an internal rumbling that there was a major life change coming. 'I was doing a lot of thinking about what my soul purpose is and what my true self is calling for. I thought I love my life here, it's so easy. I have loads of great friends, an amazing job and I'm doing great things for the community, but I feel something is missing.'

Life now couldn't be more of a contrast to how she was living for the preceding eight years. Anya had been working in the hospitality industry, travelling around the world to help restaurants become more sustainable. Being based in Bali, Indonesia, an island that is known as one of the most popular tourist destinations in the world, to now living off the land and making most things from scratch has been a surprisingly welcomed change for Anya.

Being an hour from the closest village means that Anya and her mother, who also lives at the retreat, only go to the store once a month. 'We grow most of the food for the retreats. We've planted about an acre of veggie garden and next year we have another acre to plant so we can be fully self-sufficient and not have to go to the farmers' market,' she says of their long-term dream. Growing most of their own food is a form of freedom for Anya and her family. Her goal is to get out of the system of relying on an external supply chain.

'We are learning about growing and foraging so we can always have free food – saving seeds so we don't have to buy them; keeping bees for honey if we want something sweet.' Anya feels that if they keep continuing in this way of self-sufficient living, everything will snowball.

Anya comes from an alternative upbringing with her father being a yoga teacher and her mother a herbalist. She remembers living in a terrace house that had a long garden and one day her mother banned her from going into the farthest part of the garden for a month. On her sixth birthday, with her mother's hands over her eyes, she was surprised with the gift of her own garden. 'She had made an archway of climbing roses and honeysuckle and dug out a pond and lined it with crystals. There were newts and frogs and a little vegetable patch. She said to me, "Anya this is your magic garden. You can grow food or flowers here; you can have friends here or you can say that you don't want anyone here. This is your space".' Since Anya fell pregnant with a daughter, she made plans for passing this ritual down.

Her hope for sharing her garden and natural spaces with her daughter is one she also has for the wider community. The approximately 4000 acres of land Meadowsweet Retreat lives on was once, prior to the 1950s, a whole village of crop sharers – people who would swap produce and live sustainably. Anya has begun to reinvigorate this ethos by inviting volunteers to engage in skillsharing such as mushroom foraging and beekeeping, and even inviting potters who use the natural clay from the river.

All guests are also encouraged to participate in rewilding practices during their stay. 'The guests have to come back to nature; they have to come and do a session on permaculture or forage for wild medicine. We get them into the earth and their hands in the soil. They all eat from the land while they are here and drink from the spring. That's the goal of Meadowsweet Retreat: to touch as many people's lives with nature as we can.'

Anya is deeply passionate about the retreat because she wants more people to feel the freedom of self-sufficiency and the healing potential of nature. 'I find so much peace and healing in nature. If I've had a long computer day, an argument, or am feeling overwhelmed with what's going on in the world, I can just go and spend some time in the garden – planting some seeds, digging things up, weeding – it's the best therapy. You can really work through things when you're in the quiet presence of Earth.'

'Probably the most important thing that human beings can do now is try to understand that we are just the same as an olive tree or a calendula flower. We are made of the same stuff.'

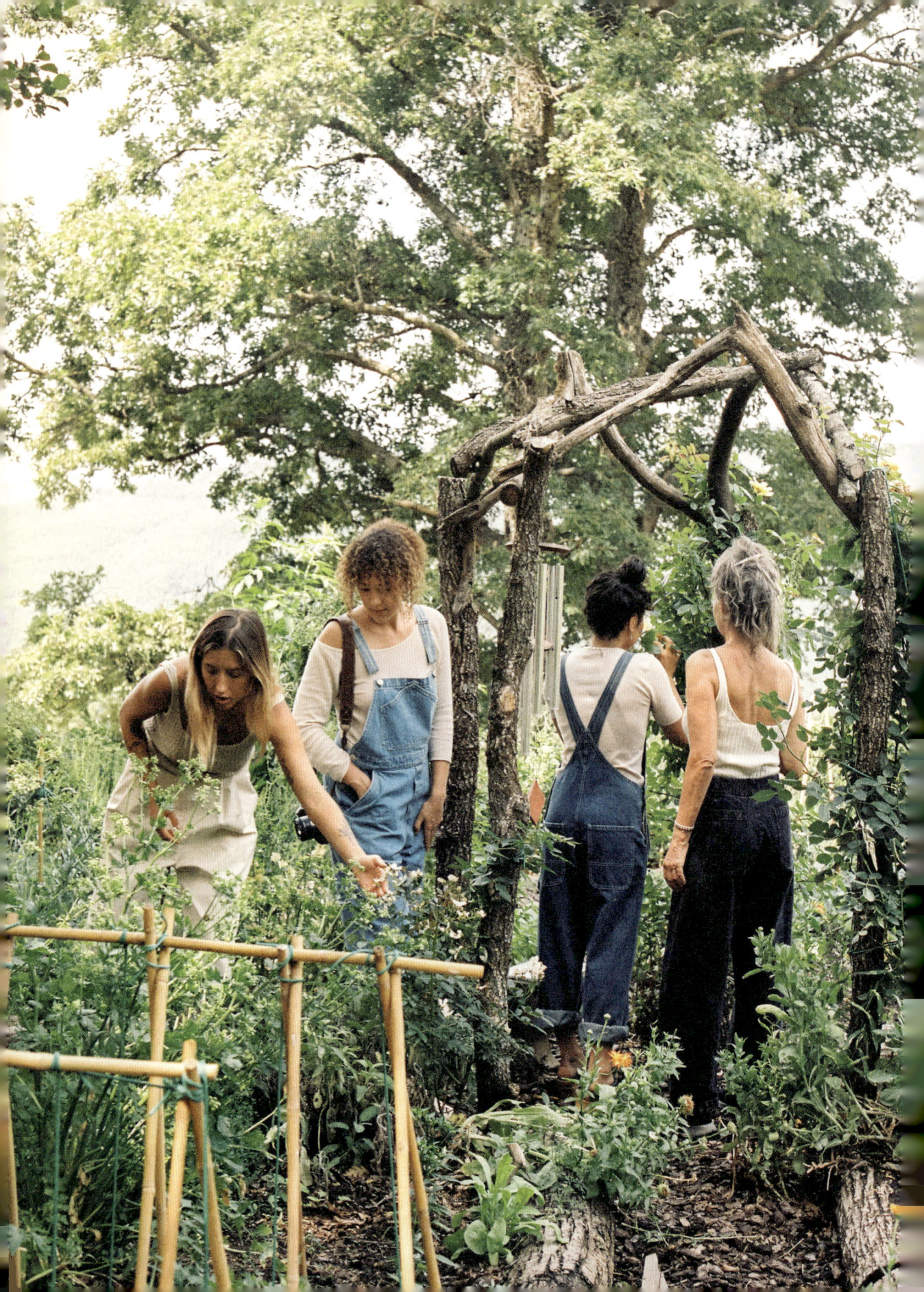

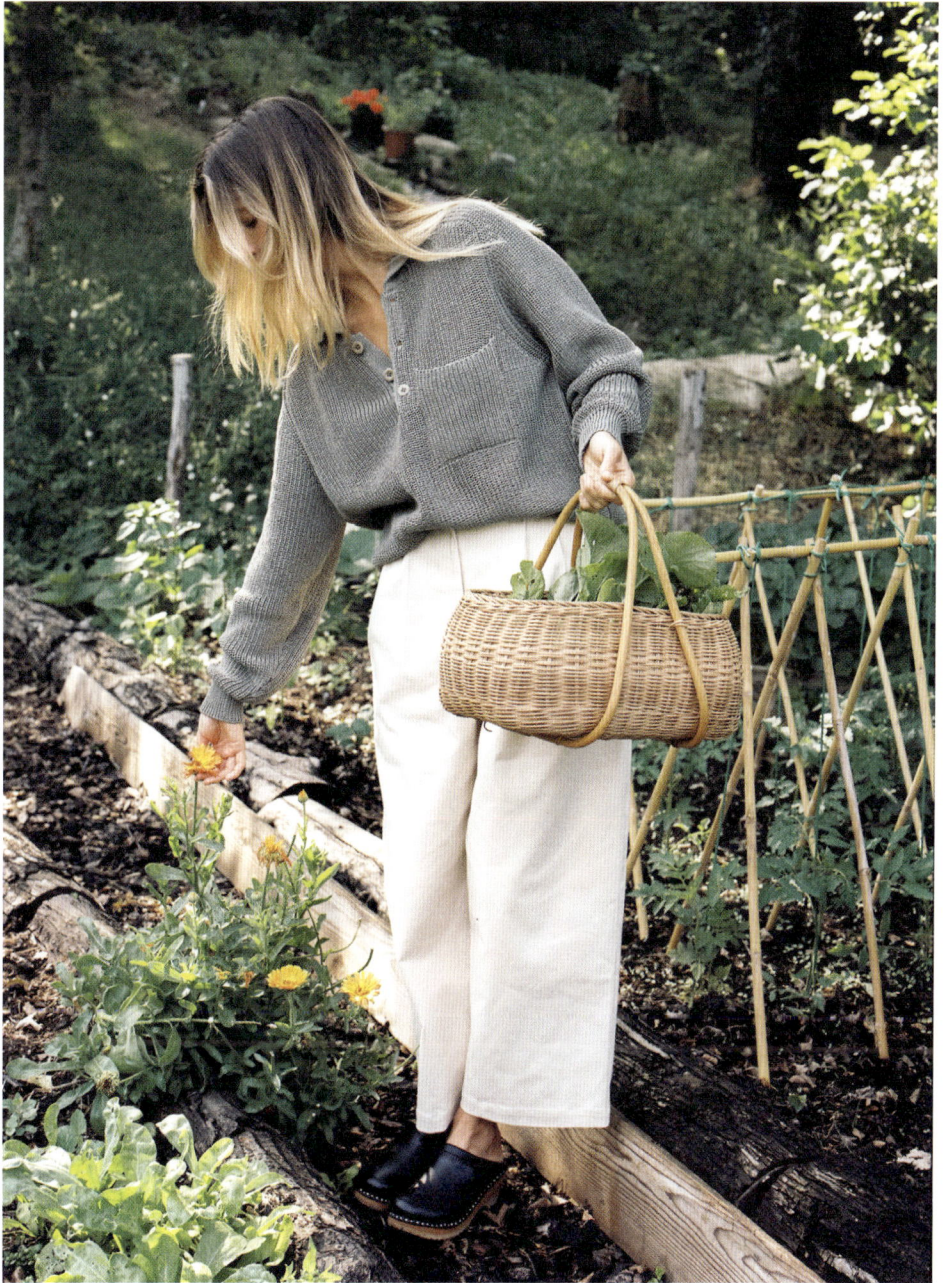

Meadowsweet Retreat offers a rewilding live-in experience for guests to realign with nature.

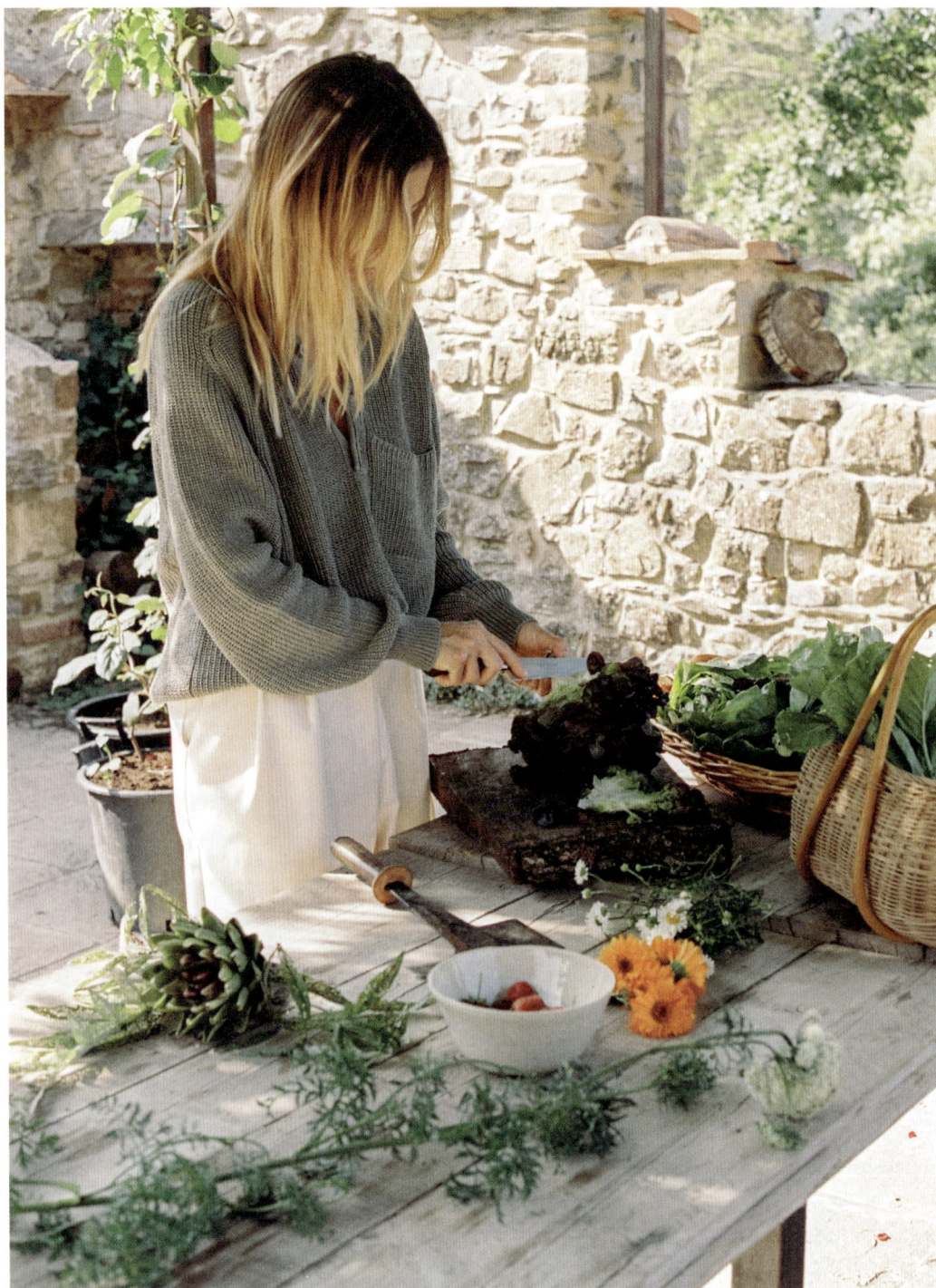

The wisdom of nature

◇ 'I find so much peace and healing in nature.
You can really work through things when you're in
the quiet presence of Earth.' – Anya Lily Montague

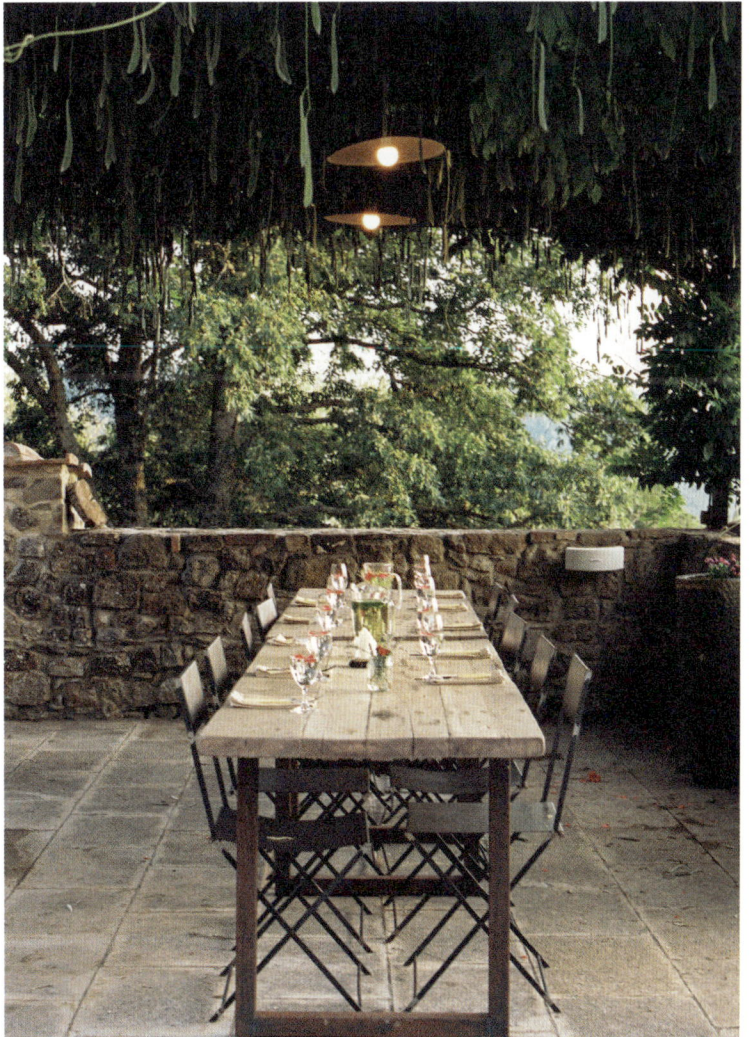

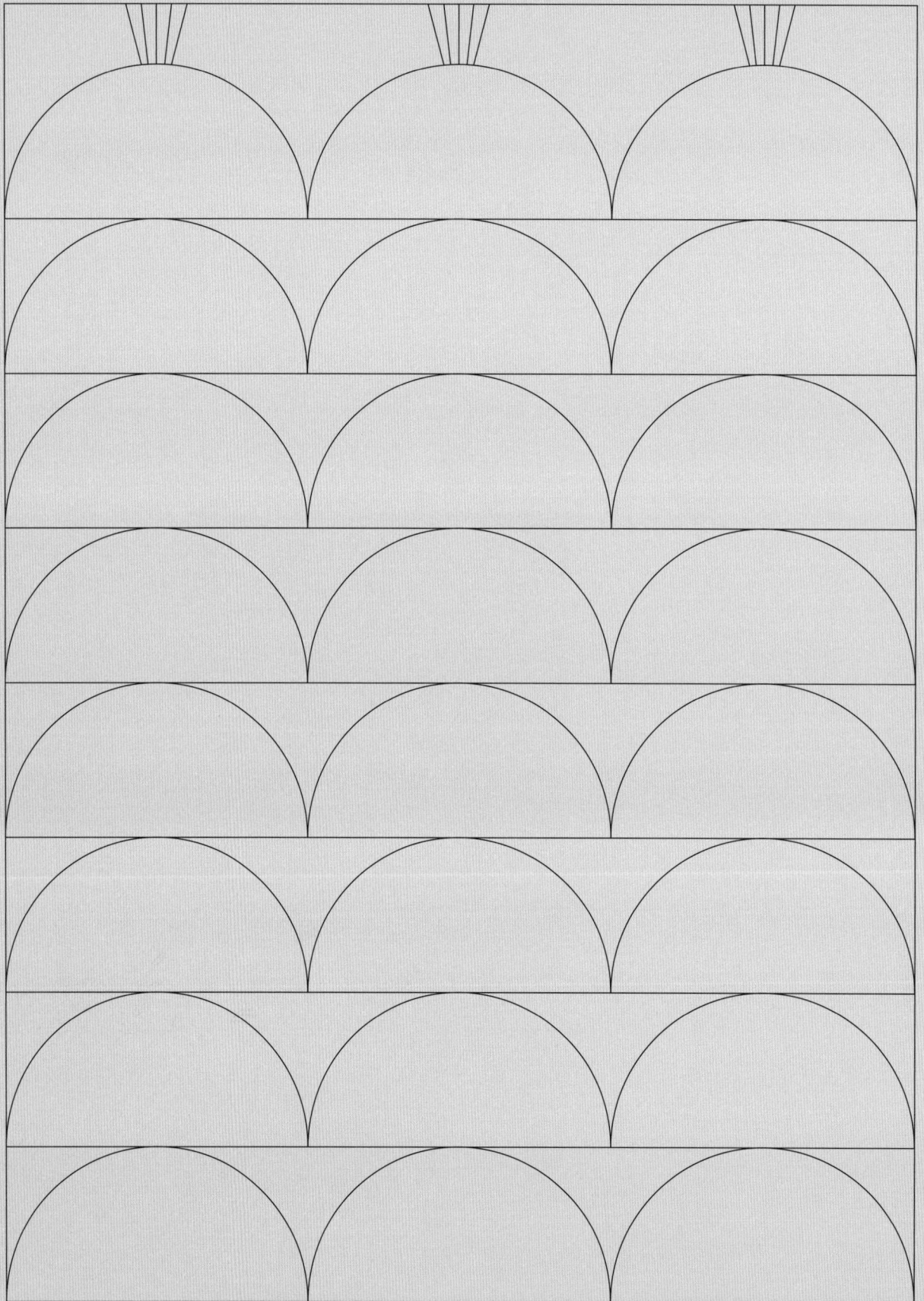

Veggie scrap broth
for reducing waste

Inspired by Anya Lily Montague

Food accounts for tonnes and tonnes of waste every day. Not only is this devastating for our fellow humans who don't have access to nutritious food, but also to the planet. It's horrifying to see the resources required to grow produce at a large scale only for it to be thrown into the bin as rubbish. In Western countries, many are particular about the parts of the produce they use, discarding undesirable organs of meat, misshapen fruits or vegetables that are bruised or a bit limp. We should balk at the waste.

Eating vegetables is one of the easiest ways we can have a relationship with nature. Even if you live in a city with limited garden spaces and you have to purchase all of your food from a supermarket, most of us can still include vegetables in our diet. I tell my patients to aim for a variety of textures and colours as much as possible, so they have the best chance of receiving the benefits such as:

- increased range of nutrients
- diversified gut bacteria
- supported immune system
- boosted energy levels
- aided digestion.

As a way to reduce your food waste and to include more vegetables in your diet, I recommend getting into the habit of making a veggie scrap broth. By boiling down vegetable scraps you are extracting the remaining nutrients into the broth before throwing them away. Not only can this be used as a stock for soups or stews, but you can drink it as an afternoon pick-me-up alternative to a cup of tea or coffee. The flavour tends to be sweet but of course changes depending on which vegetables you use and how you season it.

$\longrightarrow$

To begin ●

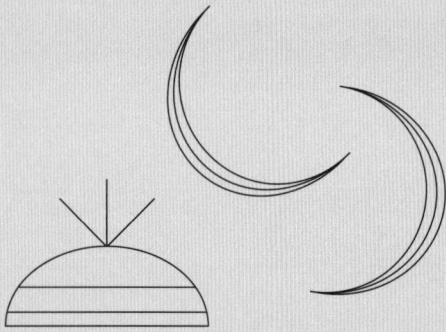

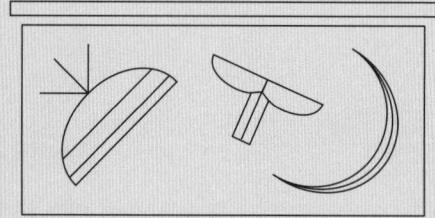

● 1
Over the course of a week or two, start collecting the off cuts of your vegetables when preparing meals. It may be the heads of carrots, the skins of onions or the cores of capsicums. (Most vegetable scraps are fine to include, however, broccoli and cabbage can have a slightly bitter taste when boiled. Do not keep or include mouldy or rotten food, no amount of boiling will get these ones back!)

● 2
Keep the scraps in a container in the freezer until you have collected about 2–3 cups worth.

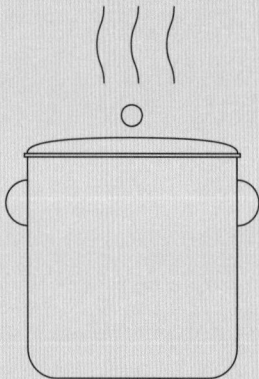

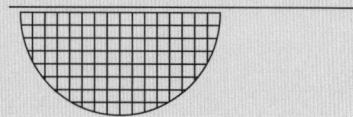

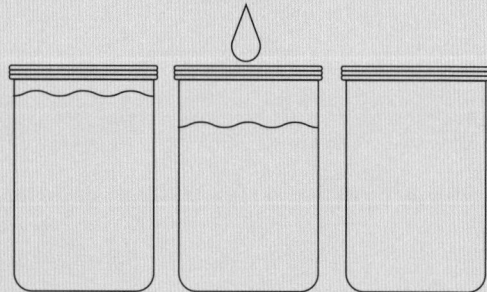

● 6
Once the broth has come to a boil, switch off the heat and let the contents cool down with the lid on.

● 7
Once the broth has cooled down, strain the liquid into clean air-tight jars or containers.

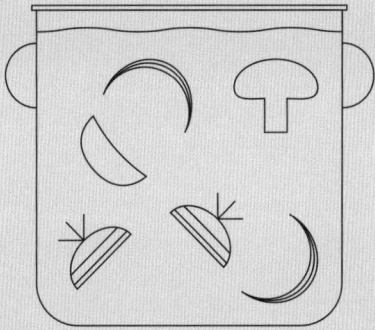

● 3
Once you have enough frozen scraps, add them to a large pot and fill with filtered water.

● 4
If you like, you can add whole garlic cloves, dried herbs or dried mushrooms for taste.

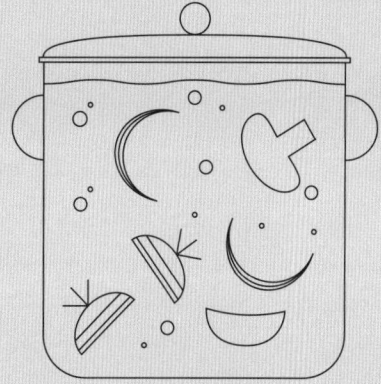

● 5
Cover with a lid and bring the contents of the pot to a slow boil on the lowest heat.

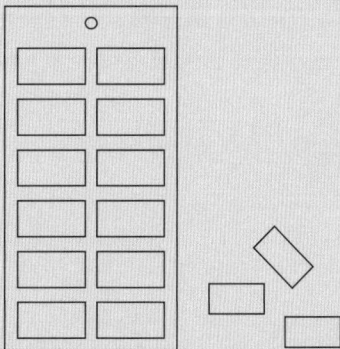

● 8
Keep your containers in the fridge and use the broth within the week. Alternatively, you can freeze the broth in ice trays to defrost and add to your meal at a later date.

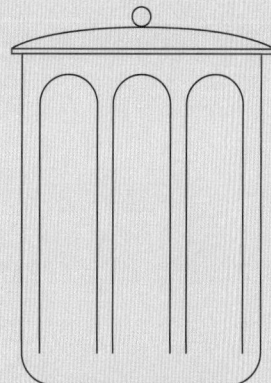

● 9
The boiled-down veggie scraps can now either be discarded in your green waste bins or added to compost.

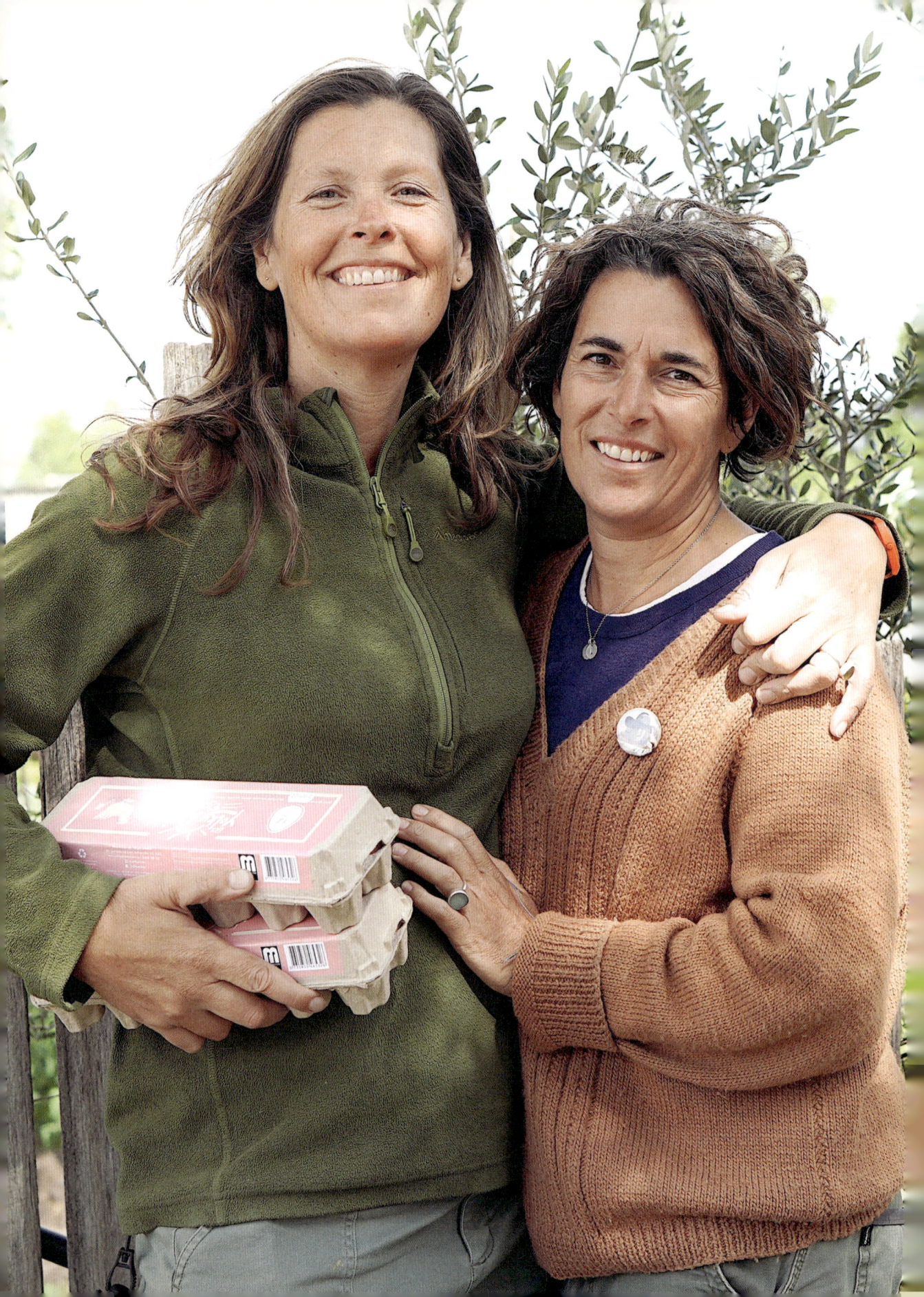

Farming

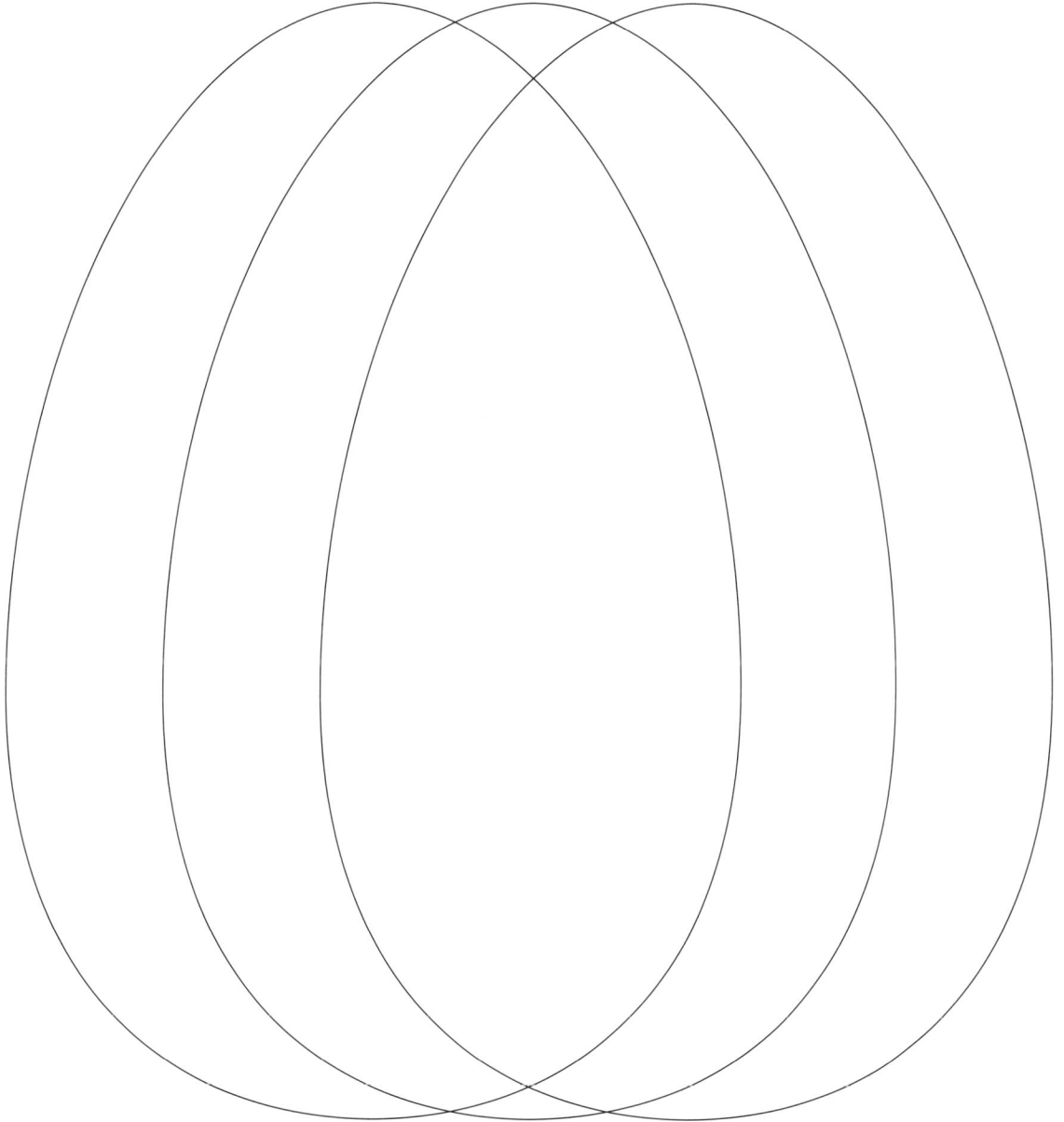

Finding emotional support from animals and the elements

Jacqui Lanarus and Gab Banay

● Australia

After Jacqui's daughter Lily was tragically killed in a four-wheel driving accident just before her 21st birthday, Jacqui and her partner Gab decided to honour her life by ticking off an item on Lily's bucket list: starting a sustainable free-range egg farm. Having no experience in farming, both women quit their jobs, bought some chickens and started collecting eggs on some land they leased near their home in Victoria, Australia.

Starting their business, lovingly called Lil's Yolky Dokey Eggs, was a way for Jacqui and Gab to heal. 'Doing thirteen-hour days in all types of weather was very difficult to start with, but I've felt that being out in nature and among our livestock and beautiful dogs has helped my healing process. I could not have gone back into an office – I wouldn't function in that space. Being out in nature was a way of being able to get by every day,' says Jacqui.

Both women have used the farm and change of environment as a way to grieve Lily. For the first few months having that space is what kept them going, whether it was used for going down to a back paddock to scream or sitting in stillness together. Gab also credits their six Maremma sheepdogs and the nearly 2500 chickens that keep them busy as a big part of their healing process. 'They really are the heart of our business and they have given so much back to us,' she says.

At the start of their farming journey, they were getting up before sunrise every morning for Lily, however, over the years their purpose has evolved to one that is centred around being part of the local food system and supplying their community with a good-quality product. As somewhat of a novelty to the people driving by, Jacqui and Gab have found great joy out of the reactions to their pasture-raised chickens. 'People couldn't stop laughing, there is something about chickens that brings a smile to your face. You could hear little kids yelling out to the dogs as mum and dad were driving past and horns tooting and people waving with arms out the window, it was just the cutest thing ever,' says Gab.

Despite the enthusiasm from their customers, the ladies have had to defend their place in the local farming community with many people not taking them seriously. However, this has been the least of their worries, as Jacqui expresses, 'The biggest hurdle is that the economy isn't set up for small-scale farming. It's very difficult to do and make good money. Your product sells out every week, but the margin is small.' Even though their eggs are a 'premium product' and the retail price is higher, running a truly sustainable free-range egg farm is not a lucrative business. The ladies have had to supplement their income by renting out a studio at their home.

Regardless of the challenges, Jacqui and Gab have found a wonderful support system in the fellow female farmers of the area. 'The women that we know in our community are brainstorming and troubleshooting and sharing how to move forward, kick goals and support one another,' says Gab. The land they are leasing in Main Ridge, Victoria, is shared with two other female producers thanks to their landlady who is trying to create opportunities for people to get into farming, a path that is traditionally inherited down the familial line.

The wisdom of nature

To see her dream come to fruition would likely make Lily very happy. Described by her mum as an oxymoron, Lily had two sides to her personality that have been woven into the farm. 'She was very glamorous and a beautician, but she also worked at a hardware store. She was very down-to-earth, on weekends she would go camping and four-wheel driving, and unfortunately that's where we lost her, but she was with her friends and she was enjoying life at the time so that's a positive,' says Jacqui.

Lily's vivaciousness has become part of the pink and yellow branding of the Yolky Dokey Eggs. Gab and Jacqui also credit the colour of sunsets as another important part of their healing process. 'Those colours came to epitomise our love for Lil and it became the colours of our Yolky Dokey cartons. We constantly had sunset-coloured flowers at home and we planted out a garden in those colours with lots of roses, perennials and fruit trees,' says Gab.

It is a sense of awe that kept the women going during the toughest months. Working long hours meant that they got to witness every sunrise, every sunset, every full moon and every rainbow. Both are endlessly appreciative of their farm, their animals and the community for supporting this journey. 'There will be days where the wind is howling, chickens are flying left, right and centre and the rain is coming down sideways. You're trying to get the eggs in before it all gets too bad or something major happens. But then all you need is one email or one phone call to say these are the best eggs I've ever eaten and it makes it all worth it,' says Gab.

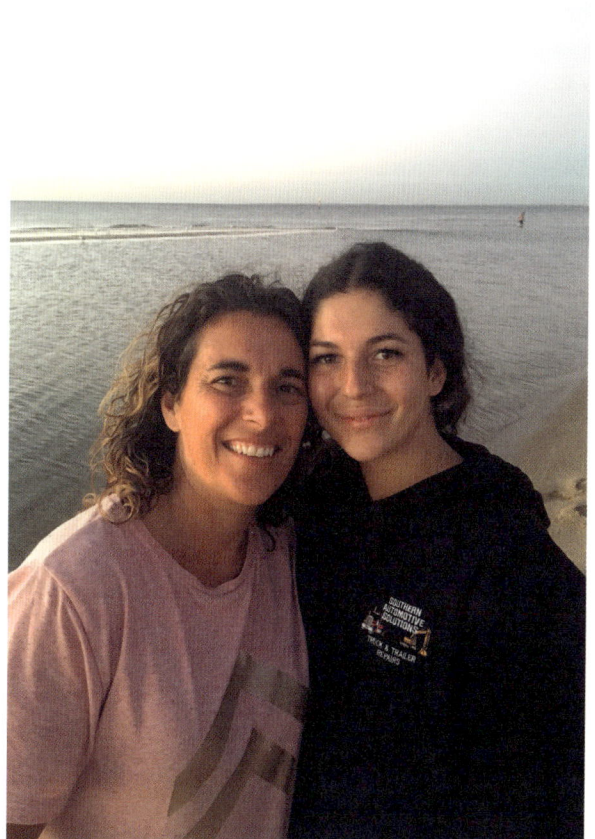

'The constant change and movement of the seasons coming and going, that has given us the energy to keep going.' – Gab Banay

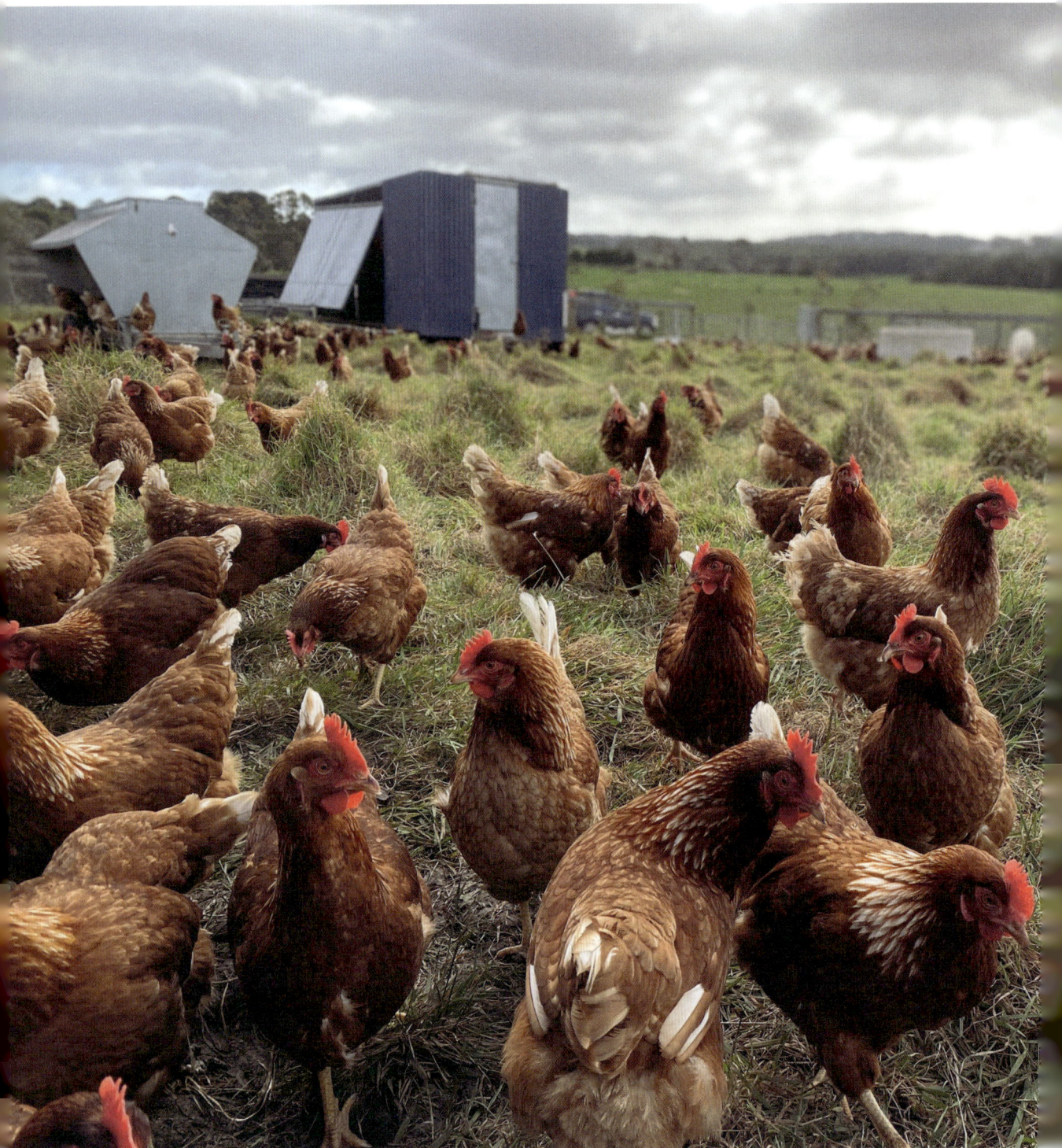

The wisdom of nature

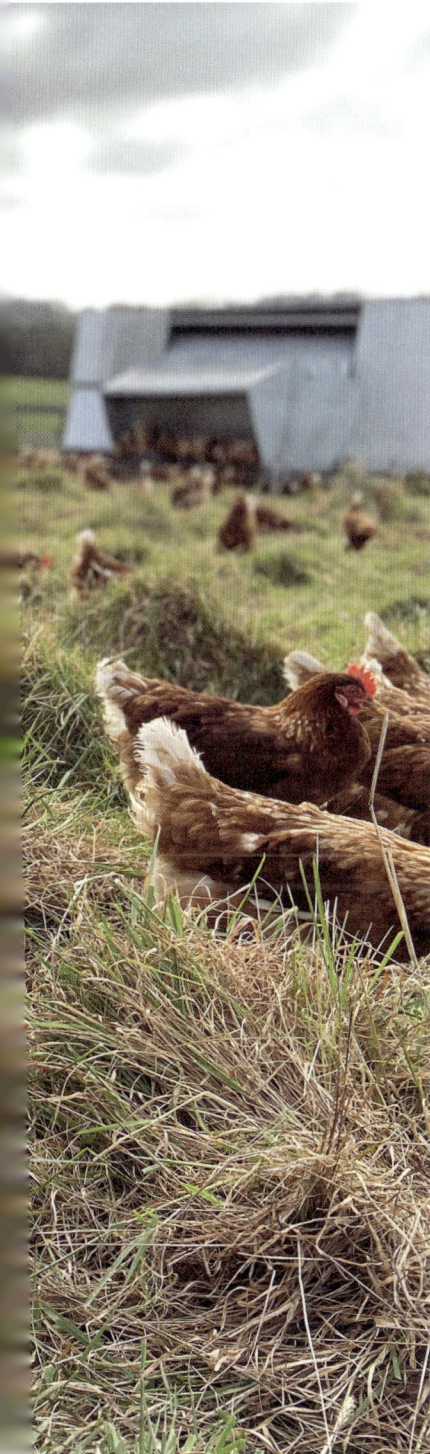

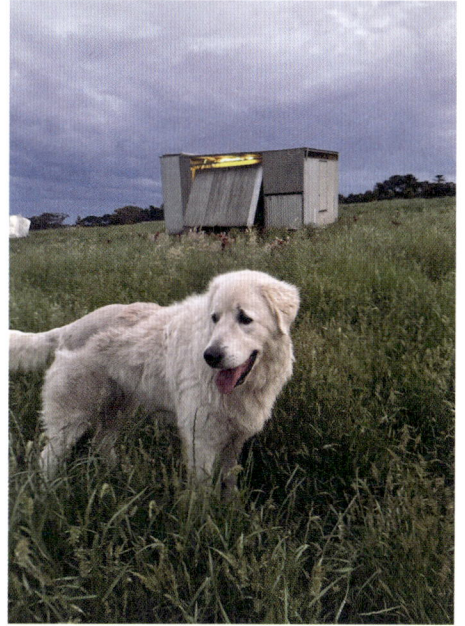

'It has been such a blessing being at the farm surrounded by nature and animals. I don't know how we would have got through it any other way.'

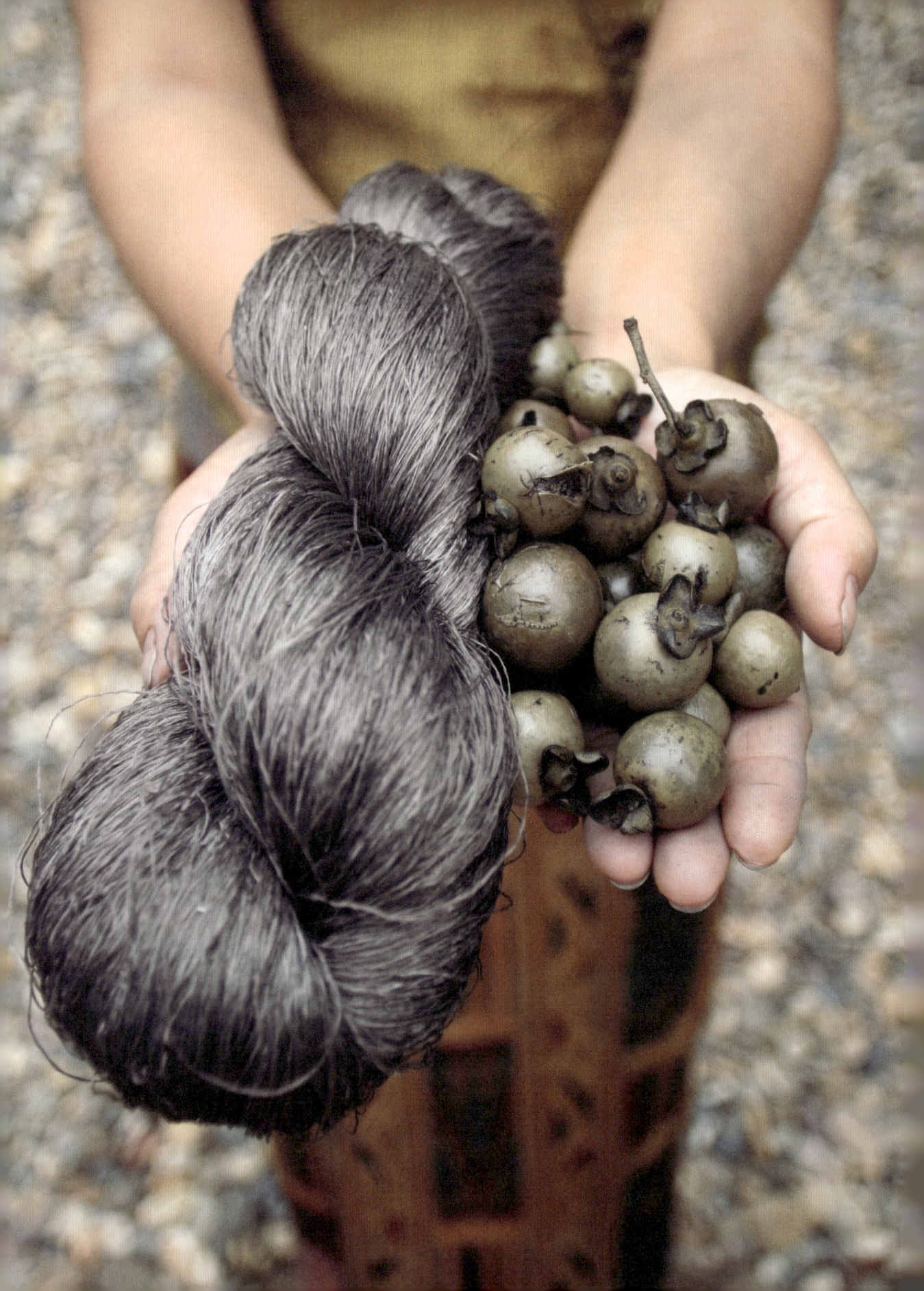

Textile design

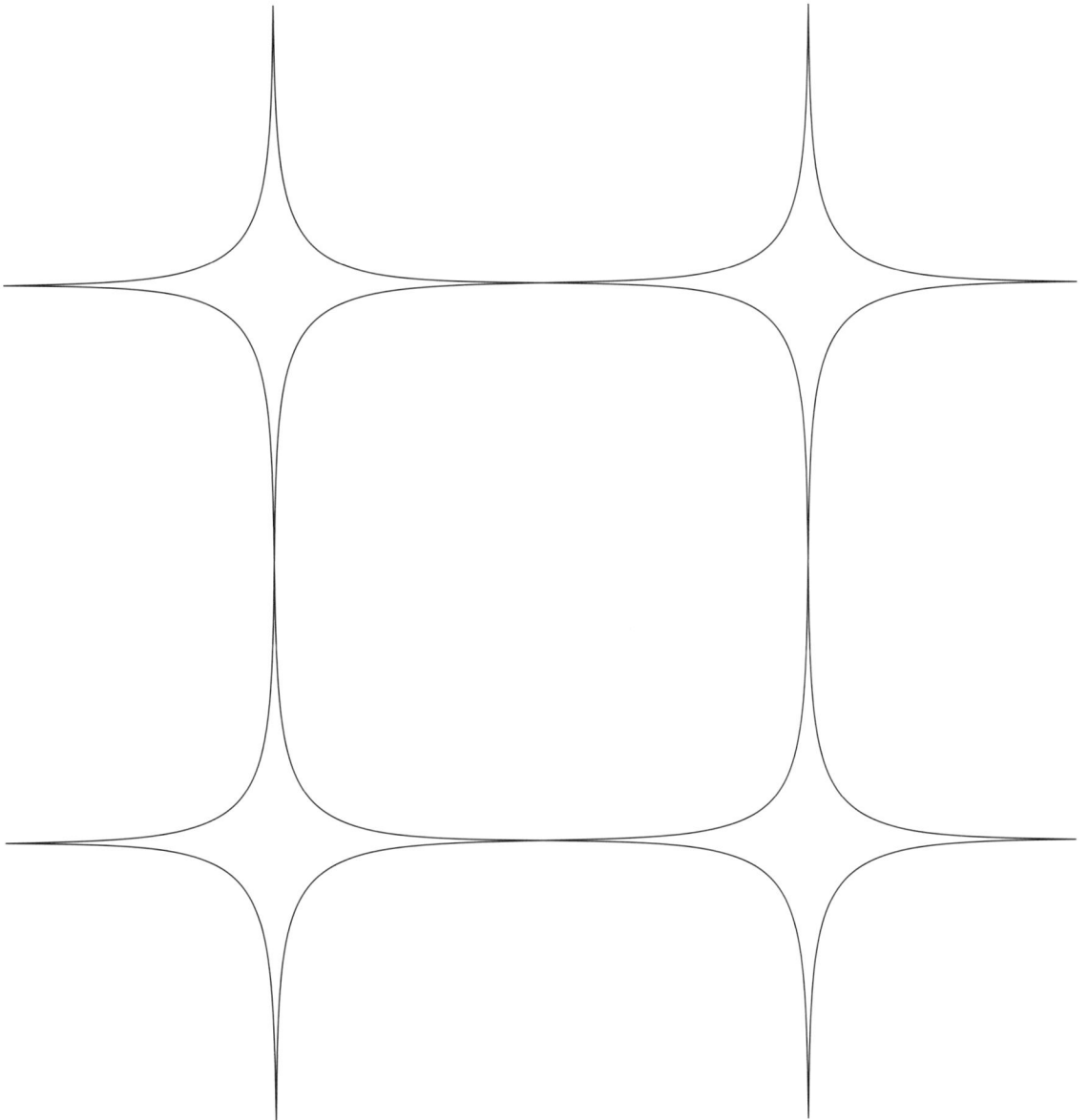

Empowering others with traditional crafts

Samorn Sanixay

● Australia

'When you learn about what's edible and what can be used for shelter, you can survive anywhere.'

Samorn Sanixay had no idea that returning to the region her family was from would eventually inspire her to create a successful textile business as well as help hundreds of women improve their quality of life. Her work is now showcased in galleries and magazines across the world, but it is the opportunity to help women thrive that is her true motivator.

Samorn was born in Laos in the early years after the Vietnam War but, as a baby, went to Australia with her family as refugees. With her mother's illiteracy and her father working day and night to provide for her and her three sisters, Samorn studied overtime to get a good education and in time went to university to study political science, human resources and languages – learning skills that would prove invaluable down the line in her work.

Initially starting out as a translator and English teacher in South-East Asia, Samorn eventually worked for the United Nations Children's Fund (UNICEF) as a researcher for books to support young girls and women with education and equality. She thought it was perfect as she considered how her mother never had the opportunity to go to school. Then by chance, when on assignment in the remote villages of Laos, Samorn came across women who were weaving. 'I thought this is really incredible, this is how they make cloth. They make it all by hand because it's so remote there.'

On her return to the city, Samorn observed how disadvantaged girls and women were directed into trades such as hairdressing or computer skills by Western Non-Governmental Organisation (NGOs) rather than being given the chance to practise their traditional crafts. Speaking with these women, Samorn realised many of them had wonderful textile skills and so, before returning back to Australia, she set up a weaving and boarding house for these women.

And thus, Eastern Weft was born, an initiative integrating the traditional weaving skills of South-East Asian women with designs catered towards a Western audience. Within a month Samorn managed to sell out their first collection by door knocking on shops in Sydney. This gave these women in Laos a wage comparable to that of a Laotian government officer. Over the years, their pieces and naturally dyed fabrics have become sought after, showcased in the Branly Museum in Paris, France, and used by renowned fashion designer Akira Isogawa.

Samorn has also set up studios in Australia to encourage local artists to practise their crafts and to teach refugee women new skills. For the year of 2022, Samorn's focus had been travelling around Australia, cataloguing and documenting over 300 species of Eucalyptus. 'Part of the fellowship is reconnecting everyday Australians with some of the uses and importance of eucalypts because every single one of us has access to them. You can print with them, you can dye with them and some of them are edible,' she says with reverence for this common tree.

It's not only the women in the weaving houses that are benefiting from Samorn's work but also the women in Australia who come to her natural-dye workshops. 'I'll never forget the time someone attended one of my classes where I talked about how rust is a modifier that shifts colour and they asked, "where would I find it?" I thought, where have you been? Rust is absolutely everywhere.' Samorn now understands that focusing her workshops on natural materials and how they can be used for dyes and for making things has helped to open many eyes.

Samorn also often reflects on some of the women in her workshops who come from privilege and have successful careers but are struggling with their worth. 'I found that incredibly fascinating,' she says, 'they're well educated, they've got money, but they have low self-esteem. It is this other aspect that I never thought about. I get to give them a craft, something to take their mind away.' Teaching women new skills and how to trust their intuition has always been an integral part of the work Samorn does.

Outside of running Eastern Weft, Samorn spends most of her time in the garden and local area looking for new materials. 'All of my dyes are homegrown or foraged in the neighbourhood – local and seasonal. Half of my dyes are grown in the garden or from food waste.' That sense of wonder from nature and uncovering something new brings Samorn a sense of joy and keeps her going on this path.

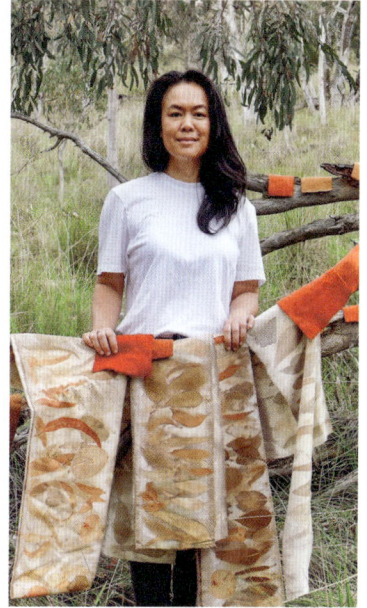

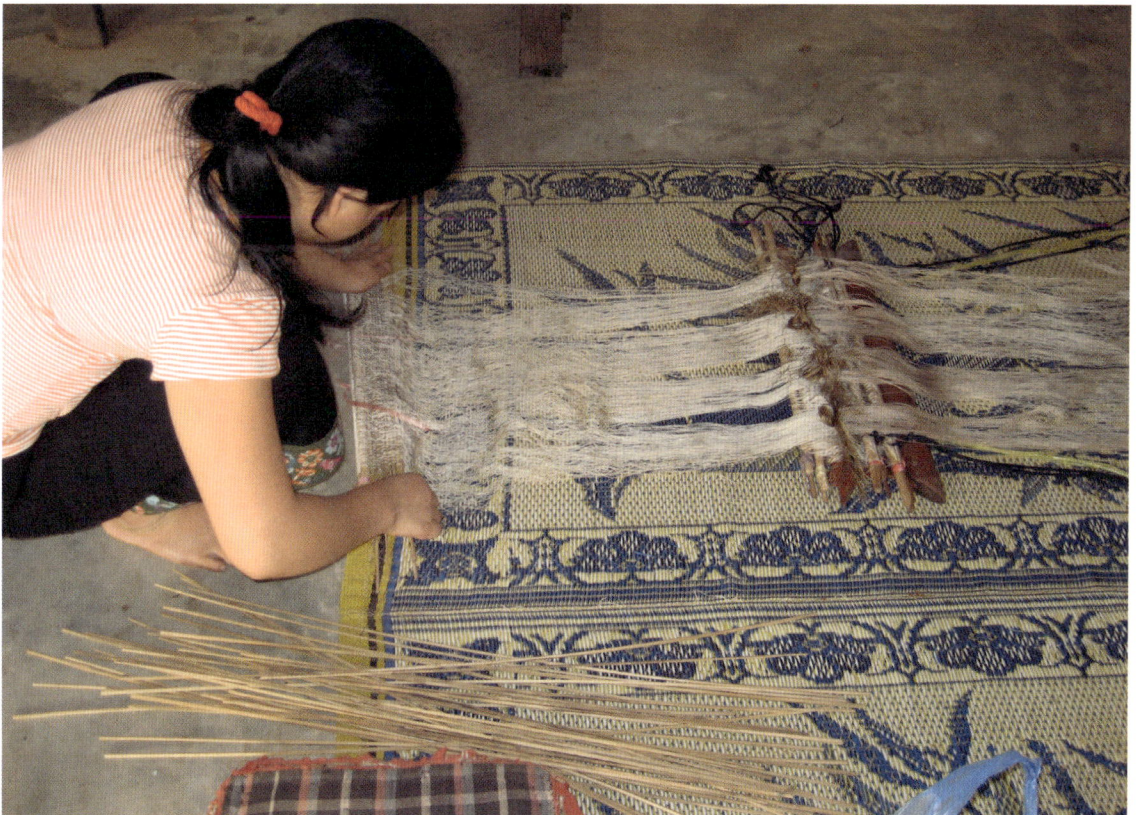

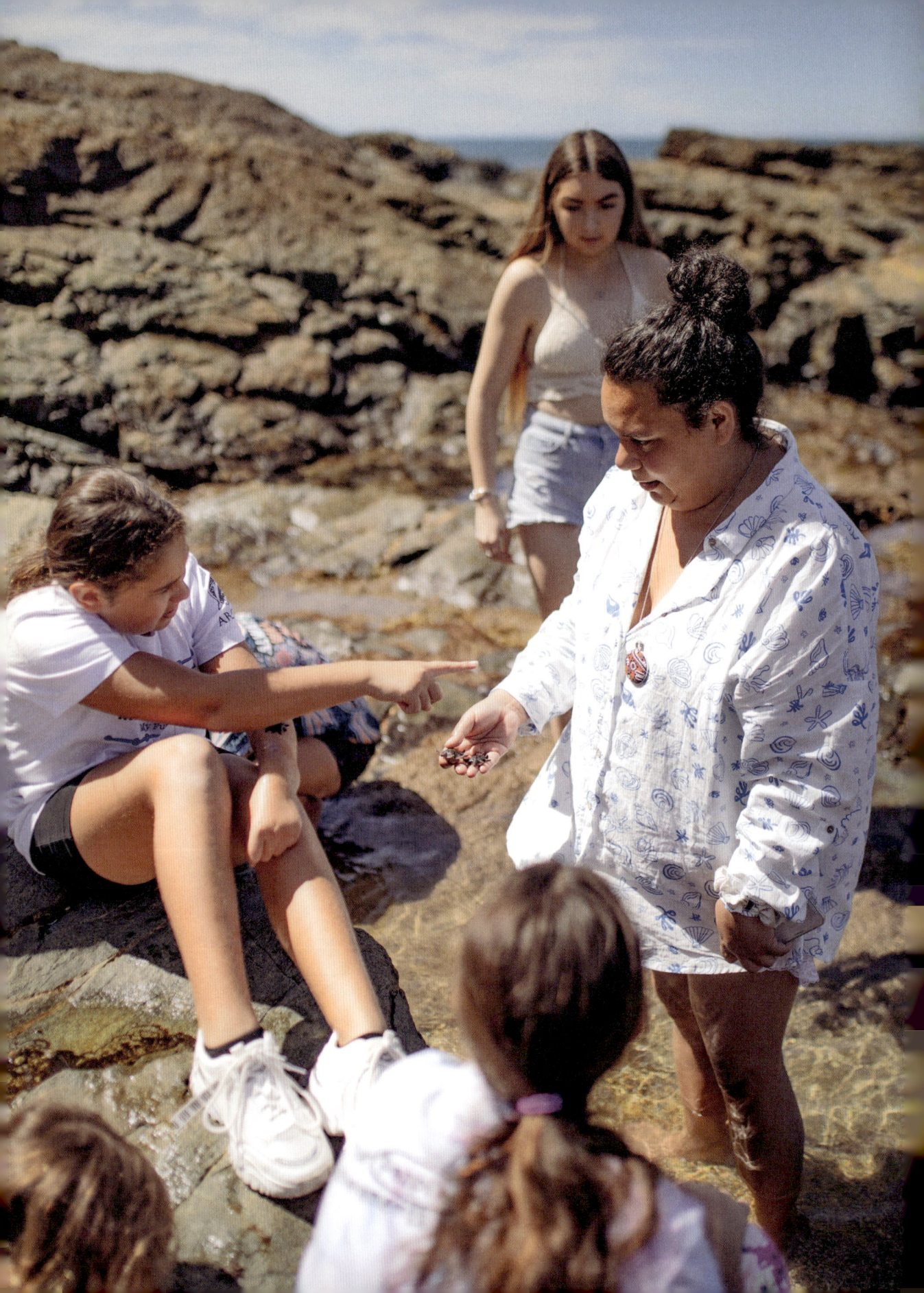

Ocean education

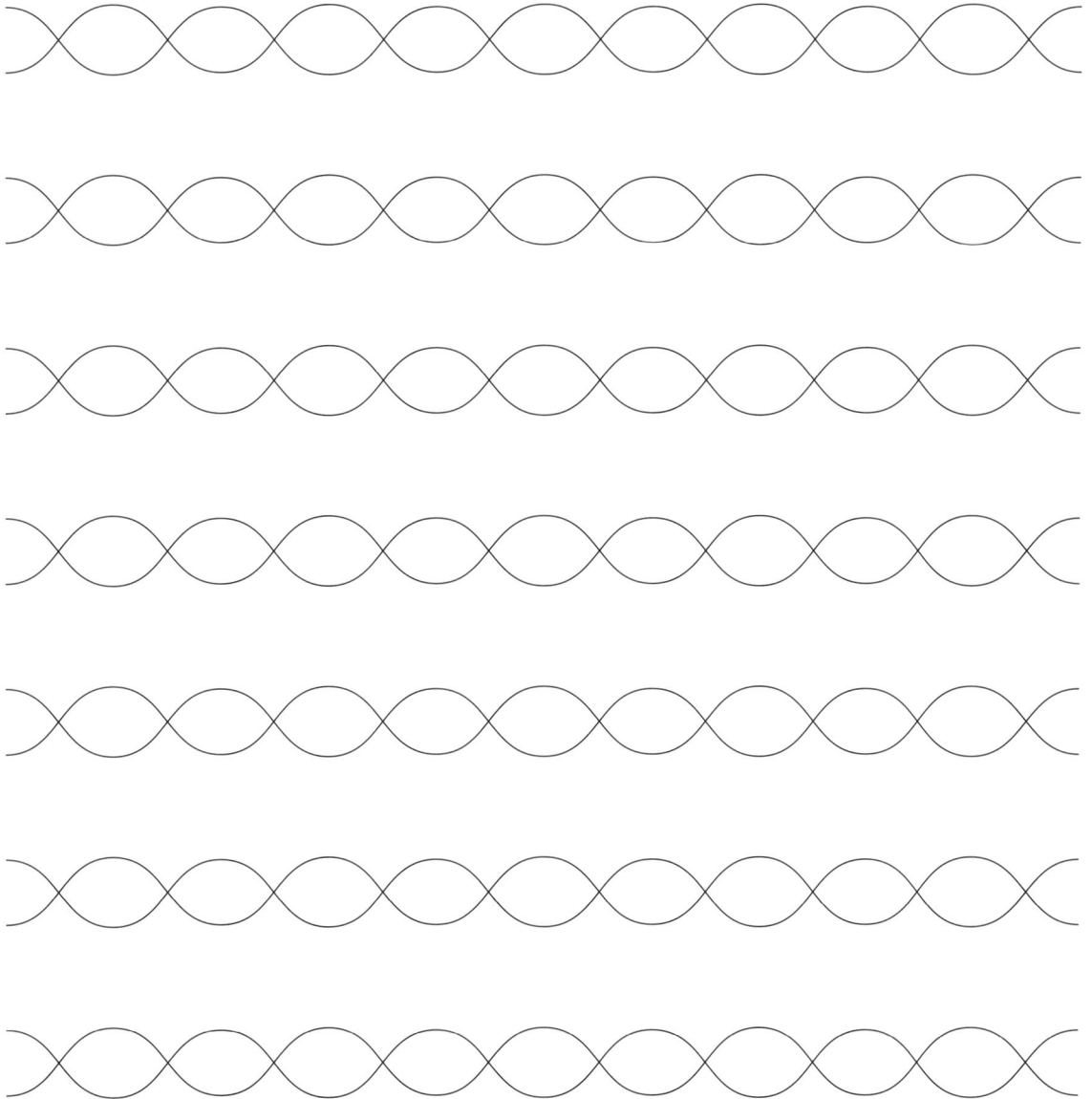

Weaving cultural knowledge into modern education

Rhiannon Mitchell

● Australia

Rhiannon Mitchell, a First Nations woman from the Mununjali people of Beaudesert in Queensland, Australia, founded her business Saltwater Sistas as a way of empowering women and young people. The business is part ocean education and part mentoring and support work. As someone who went through the legal and foster care systems herself, Rhiannon has first-hand experience that allows her to relate to many of the youth she works with. 'Before I was eighteen, I was in trouble with the police a lot. I went to many different schools and was in foster care,' she says, 'I understand what it feels like to be displaced from your family or your culture.'

Much of what Rhiannon experienced in her adolescence is what she refers to as a disconnect from her Aboriginal culture. 'Usually our problems are from the chaos of the world. Chaos can be from marriage or children, or a nine-to-five job. I think we should go back to the ways of the traditional owners of the world,' she says, 'because they were put on this planet first for a reason: to teach people how to live the right way.' While she does not think that non-Indigenous people are wrong, her belief is that we need to connect to nature and go back to a simpler way of living. 'In our culture, we have always been taught that the land is before us, that we have to protect the land and the land will look after us.'

Growing up in the small town on Gumbaynggirr Country in New South Wales, Australia, Rhiannon was always immersed in nature as a child. 'We live where the river meets the sea. It was always my happy place, a place that through school we spent a lot of time with our Elders.' Her family often went camping and, along with her siblings and friends, she was encouraged to play outdoors. However, Rhiannon does not consider her family to be as invested in the natural world as she is. 'My family loves spending time in nature, but they aren't environmentalists.'

Rhiannon's love of the ocean eventually led her to study at the National Marine Science Centre in Coffs Harbour. Unlike many of her peers, her goal is not to conduct research or work in a lab. Instead, she wants to bring her knowledge of marine biology into workshops for young people to attend so they too can foster a deep appreciation for our oceans. In late 2022 Rhiannon conducted her first six-week youth program which garnered such interest it was over-booked. The children learnt about the local reefs, endangered animals, the impacts of pollution on the ocean and traditional First Nations stories. 'Hopefully it inspires them to be the generation that looks after and protects our oceans and our land.'

Along with running more youth programs, Rhiannon has big dreams for the future. 'I'm going to get a Saltwater Sistas van so I can pick up the local girls from disadvantaged backgrounds and take them to the beach to surf and snorkel – do nature-based activities with them,' she says excitedly. Her plan is to also take the van to remote areas of Australia where communities may never have met a marine scientist before. This will give her an opportunity to exchange her knowledge on the latest research with their wisdom and stories of the environment.

This kind of knowledge exchange is something Rhiannon has sought out before when she travelled to North Dakota, USA, to spend time with a group of Native American Elders. 'They shared some really beautiful messages with me about the environment that really resonated with me,' she says, 'and many of these are the same as Aboriginal culture.' They include:

- Everyone on this Earth comes from native roots.
- If we don't take care of our mother, our animals and our spirit, our world will be destroyed.
- When we speak and stand up for ourselves, we will heal.
- Nothing starts with you. It started back with our ancestors.
- Women are sacred.

To entice women who have grown up in modern culture back into nature, Rhiannon highlights the positive impacts spending time in natural spaces has on her appearance. 'I feel beautiful in nature. I think it makes you prettier. People comment saying I look happy, and my skin looks good after I've been in nature,' she says. 'I grew up as a black big girl thinking that I had to be skinny and blonde, but when we go back to our natural selves, that's when we start to feel good.'

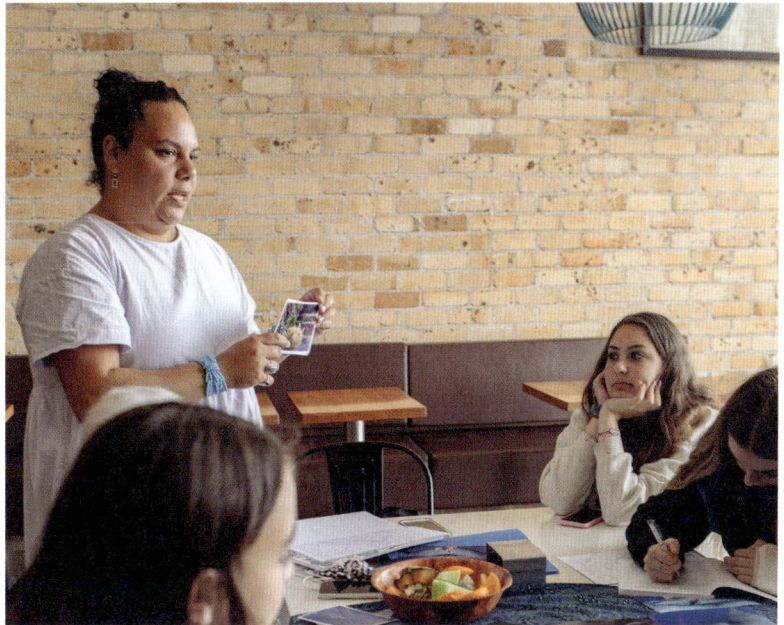

'In the morning I greet the day. I greet the Sun, the trees and the ocean. Our ancestors did this too.'

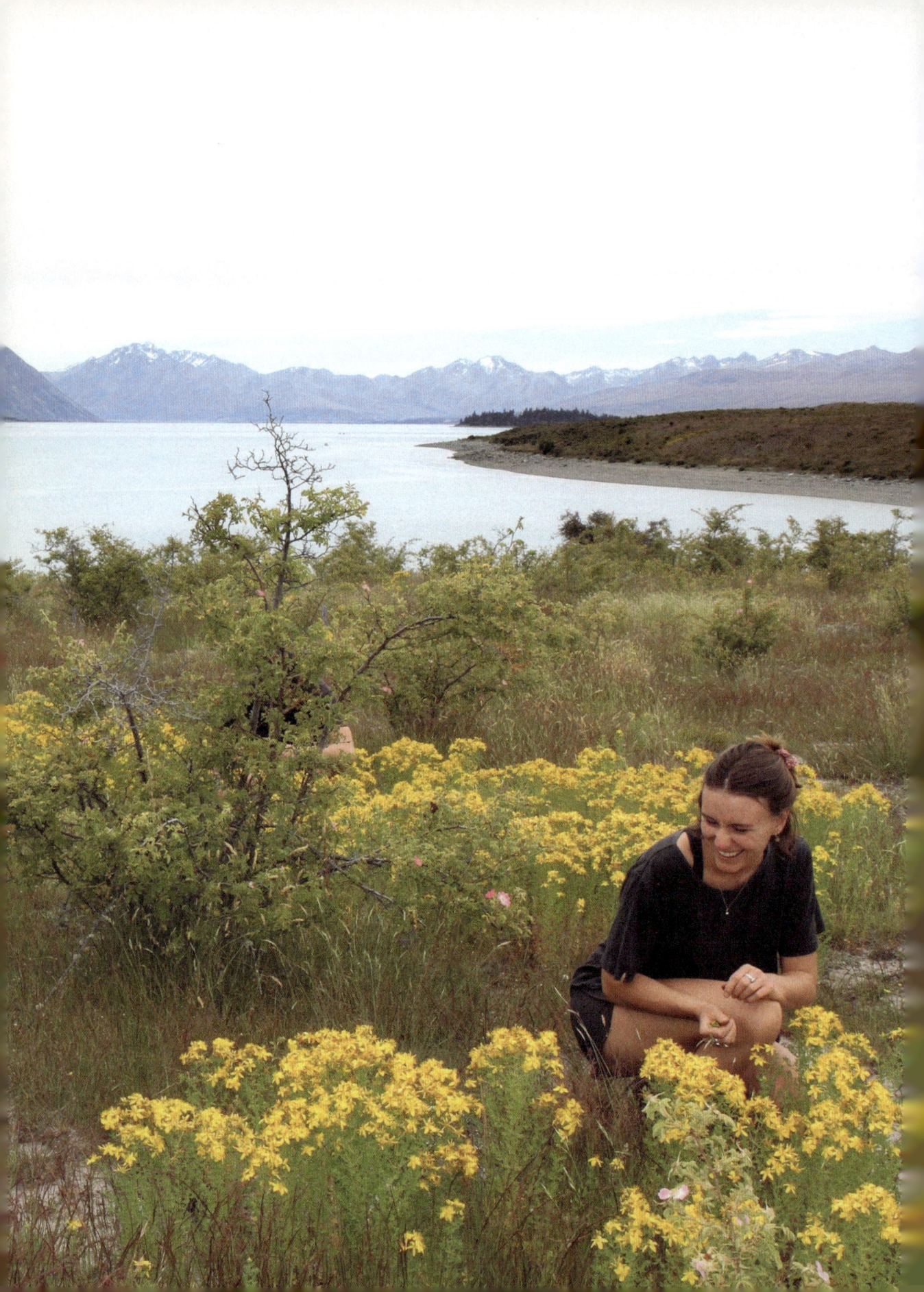

Skin care

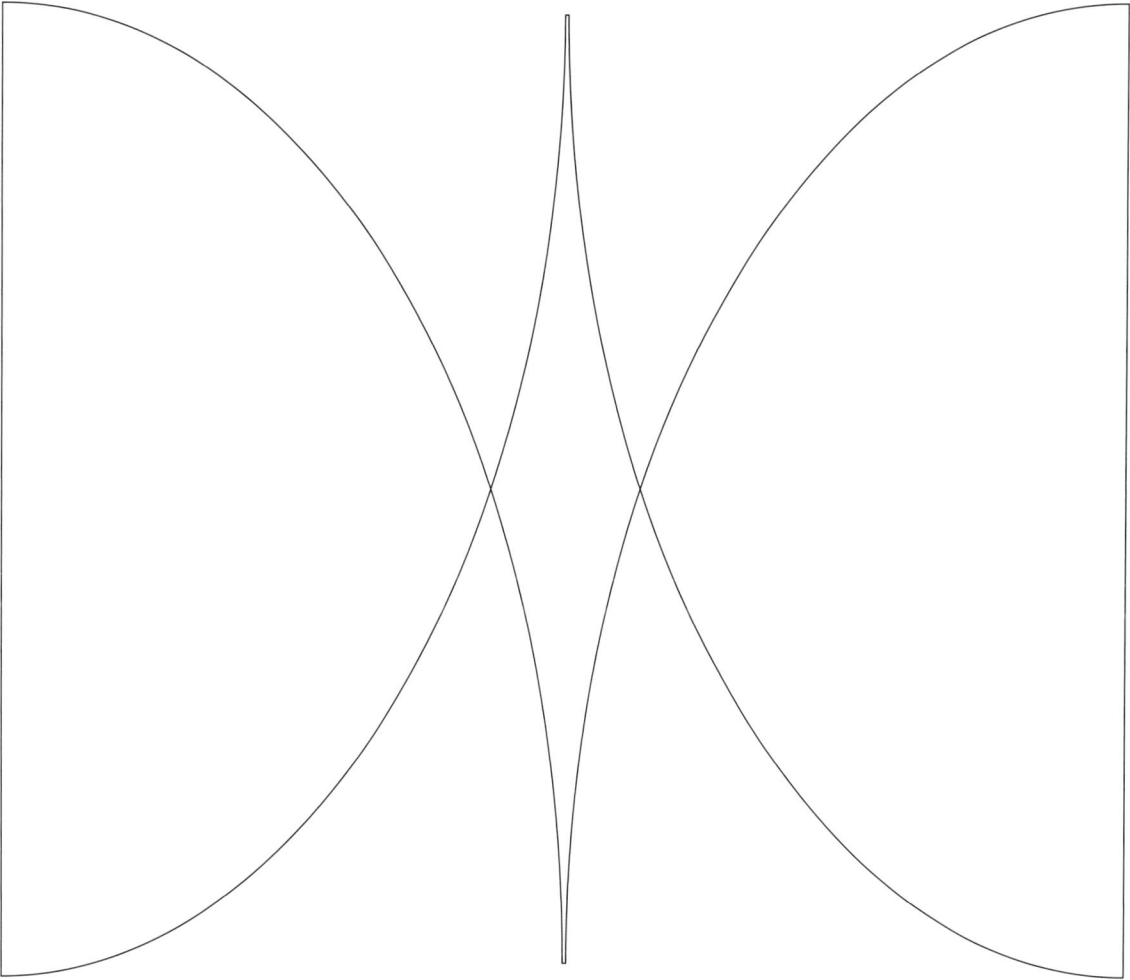

Blending nature with science

Gab Abell

● Australia

'When I work in
alignment with nature,
the flow is there;
I don't have to force
anything. It feels right
in my bones.'

Trying new things appears to be a theme throughout Gab Abell's life so far. This inquisitiveness is how she came to be on her current path as the owner and head formulator of Studium Essentials, a herbal medicine-informed skincare line based out of New South Wales, Australia.

As a young girl Gab wanted to be a wildlife videographer. 'The thing I found so enchanting about nature documentaries is seeing parts of the outside world like you've never seen before. Whether it's a frog in a little bromeliad or a bird taking flight from the nest for the first time. That's what really drew me.' However, two weeks into a degree of film and media studies at university, she knew this was not the right path for her and she made a split decision to enrol in a biomedical science subject. This eventually led Gab to naturopathy, the system of healthcare based on the power of nature, and it was the memories of her long struggle with cystic acne as a teenager that drove her to create Studium Essentials. 'Looking back, I wish I had known what to do for my skin then, but it's a blessing because it's led to where I am now. I can relate to people as I have experienced the same thing.'

Studium Essentials started off with a humble line of natural perfumes that Gab made from her bedroom but has now evolved into her full-time job. Undertaking cosmetic chemistry courses has allowed her to create a range of nature-based products that have scientific evidence behind them. 'I do lots of things to ensure there is a nice balance between the art, the spirit and the science of formulation and herbal medicine,' she says, likening the process to baking, whereby precision of temperature, measurements and time is imperative to the end results.

Gab sees skin care as a way to bring plant medicine into the mainstream. 'You can use it as a method to commune with plants that doesn't involve going to sit in a field. You can get up, have a shower and put some face oil on. It can be as simple and accessible as that.' She is often asked if her products work as well as conventional skin care because they are natural and her belief is that there isn't only one way or the other. 'There isn't a line that's drawn in the sand where there is nature and then there is science. Science is nature and nature is science.'

Gab can understand the reluctance or intimidation that some people may feel towards natural skin care and herbal medicine. She herself didn't have a lot of exposure to them growing up and admits to not even knowing what naturopathy was when she first enrolled in the course. Coming from what she describes as a conventional upbringing, she remembers an old trough in the backyard where her mum grew herbs. 'We had a pretty standard meat and vegetable diet but the fact that mum could go out and pick some parsley and put it on top of our food, I remember that memory of learning that food doesn't just come from the supermarket.'

Now in her spare time, Gab likes to hike and has recently started rock climbing. After first beginning in the local gym to learn the basics, she is now self-sufficient and confident to go on multi-pitch climbs. Gab describes climbing as the most potent form of mindfulness. 'When you are on the wall, there is no room for other thoughts. You have to be so focused and specific on where to put your feet and everything has

The wisdom of nature

to be considered.' Thanks to a robust climbing community in her area, Gab now feels the urge to give back and teach others.

This sentiment spans not only rock climbing but her work. Seeing the results of her customers is what keeps her going during times of self-doubt or the lulls of business. With this in mind, Gab continues to expand her offerings and hopes to bring the power of plants and nature to more people in the future.

'I know that what I'm practising now is from a lineage of thousands and thousands of years of women working with plants and people. It's in all of our DNA, all of our cells remember that, so I feel really privileged to carry on this tradition.'

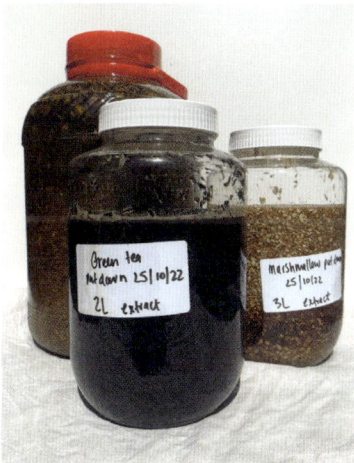

'We have evolved with plants.
It's part of our DNA.' – Gab Abell

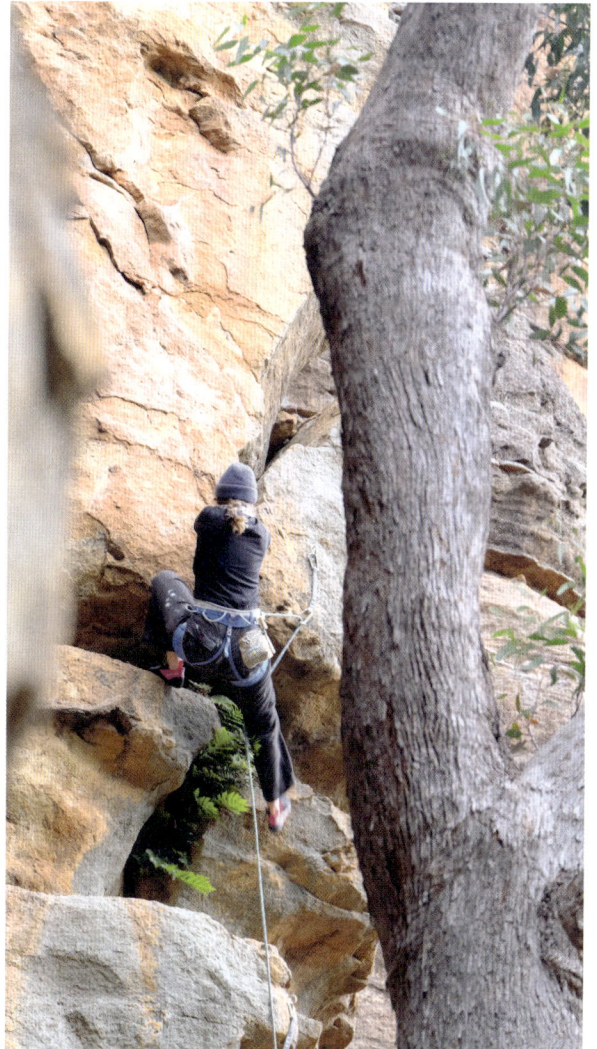

The wonder of nature

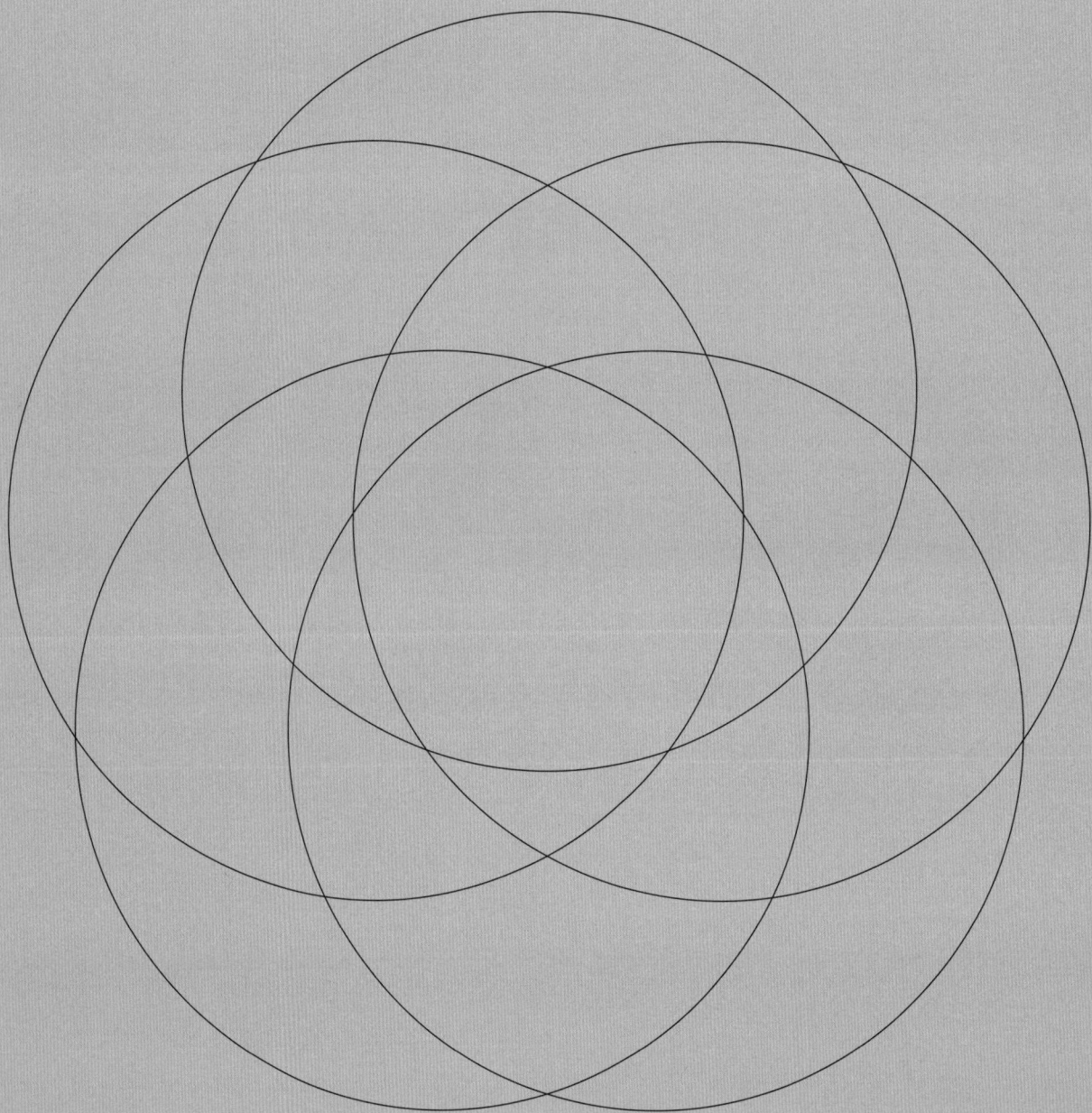

Nature has been the subject of poems, paintings and songs for as long as we have been creating. Our earliest known artworks found buried underground and on stones and caves around the world feature animals, plants and our own bodies.

I'll never forget seeing a huge whale carved into a rock when hiking in Royal National Park, Sydney, Australia. To witness the reverence of this majestic whale (burri burri in Dharawal language) and its significance to the Dharawal Aboriginal people over 2000 years ago when it was carved, helped me to realise our inherent appreciation for nature.

Wonder is more than just appreciating the usefulness of something; it is marvelling at its beauty. We don't see fireflies and think oh I wonder how I could use those for my benefit? We don't see a multicoloured sunset and think could I harvest this for my family? We don't travel far and wide to climb a mountain, look out at the view and think this is going to provide us with a roof over our head and food on our table. We do it to be a witness; to feel moved, to inspire us. We do it for the wonder.

And where does that wonder lead us? It guides us to action, to pursue our dreams, to try something new, to protect that which inspires us. The experience of wonder is what gives us hope for a brighter future.

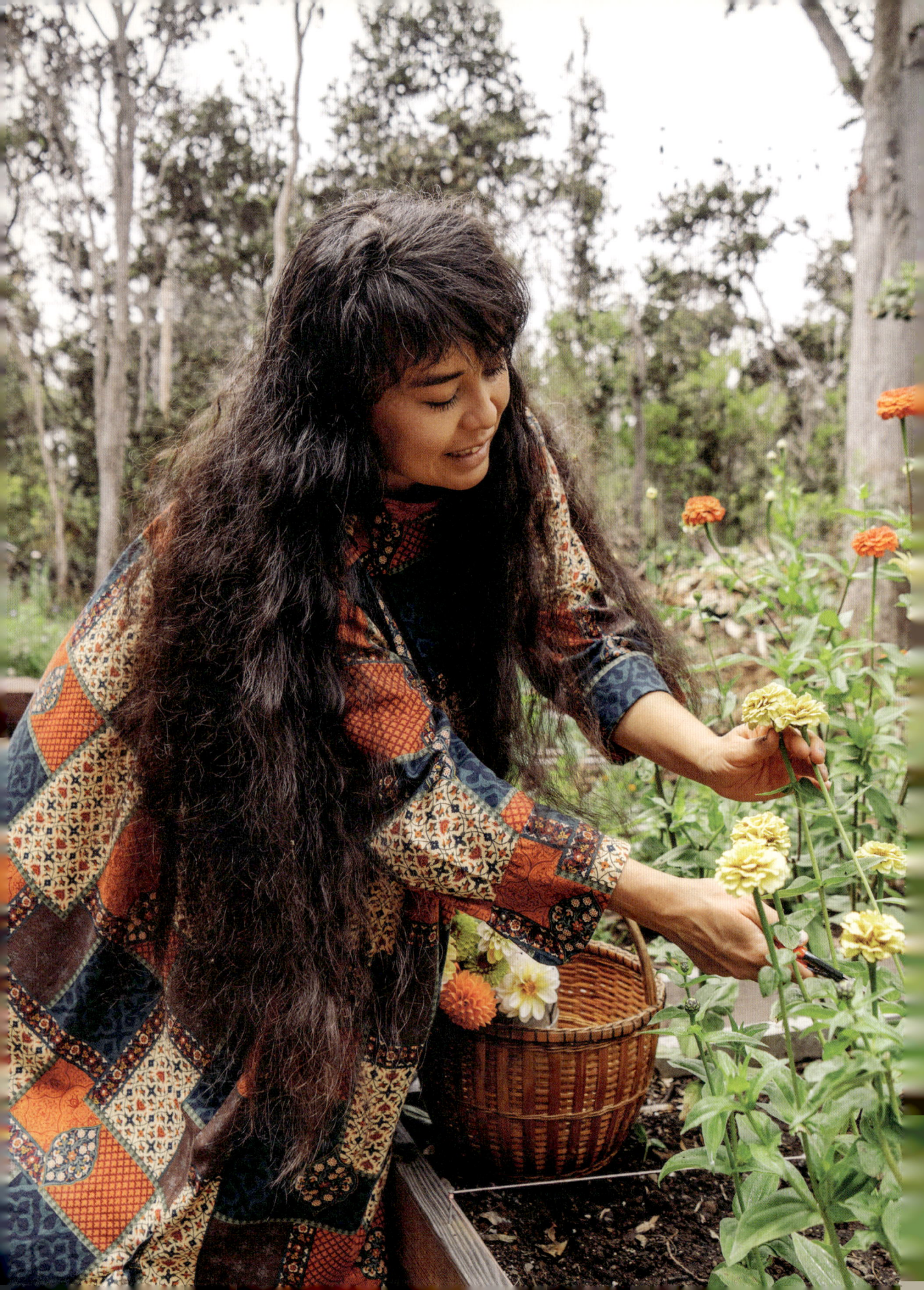

Flower growing

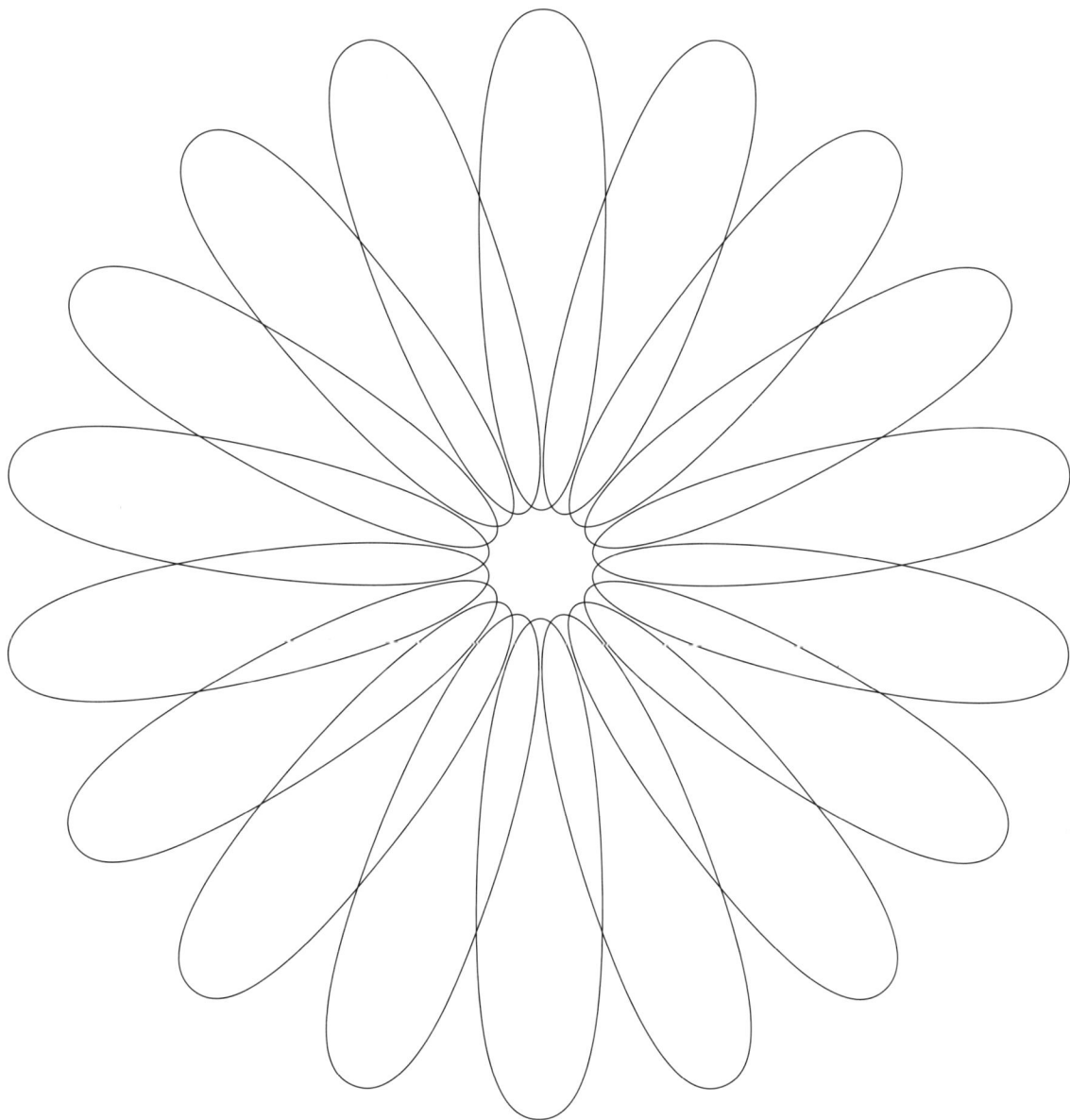

Strengthening culture with nature's offerings

Wai'ala Ahn

● Hawaii, USA

'We call her Mother Earth for a reason. When we think of her as our mother and think about what mothers really do, there is nothing that she won't do to make us better people and to help us.'

Wai'ala Ahn lives 4500 feet up the slopes of Mauna Loa, the world's largest volcano on Hawaii's Big Island. Every day she experiences earthquakes as the magma underneath the surface moves. What might be met by most people with fear, for Wai'ala it has fostered a deep reverence for the land. 'Growing up and being from this place, as well as my ancestors being from here, it's a really beautiful lesson in impermanence and being very present with what's here and what you have,' she says of this recent time of increased activity.

'We have a practice that when there are earthquakes and known activity in the area, we clean our whole house and yard, we make ourselves and our area ready for the most honourable guest. If she wants to come into our home, it is ready.'

Aside from the potential of volcanic eruption, the kīpuka (a patch of land surrounded by old lava flow) where Wai'ala's homestead is located is a welcome change from the warm beaches she grew up on. It is a place of true seasons and profound abundance. 'Our neighbours are growing things that people don't even think grow here in Hawaii, like peaches,' says Wai'ala of her close-knit community and the land around her family's home.

After studying digital design at art school, Wai'ala begun to connect more deeply to her traditional cultural practices after attending a women's gathering in California, USA. 'How I was raised was to bring gifts from the place that you're from. I made all of these leis (floral garlands) and brought them as gifts for my teachers and people I met. There was an Elder there who asked why I was not teaching this,' she says. 'I went back the next year and I think some people thought I was just going to teach them how to make flower crowns, but it was really about the interconnectedness and reverence with nature.'

During that trip, Wai'ala met someone who taught her about natural-dye making and all of the dots connected for her. 'When you undo these leis and make dye from them, then you can keep these presents and these elements with you always in a whole other form.' A practice of impermanent beauty then became a little more enduring. It was also another way to connect further with her Hawaiian heritage. 'We've had natural dyes and textile making as part of our cultural history for a long time and there are certain colours that are only found in Polynesia.'

Wai'ala's preference for dye making is with plants that are considered weeds. She prefers to give them a new meaning and to change their story from pest to precious. 'I'm learning the stories of these plants from the perspective of the people where these plants are native. There are certain plants here that are our ancestor trees and I can tell a long folklore story about them. Then I realised that's the exact same thing for these plants that have been introduced here.'

Coming from a lineage of flower growers, creating her own flower farm made sense for Wai'ala and her horticulturist husband. They decided from the get-go that they would practise a slower style of farming, where they produce less flowers than other farms and stay strong to their ethics. Seasonal, local and organic are the foundations from which their farm is built. 'Growing all together are flowers, potatoes, beets and carrots. It's not a manufactured garden at all.'

'We usually have our garden well tended except for this season – it's pretty wild. The brussels sprouts are going too far and the potatoes are peeking out. The garden and the plants are reflecting this season of our life,' she says in reference to parenting a toddler. While the garden may seem chaotic, witnessing her son building a relationship with these plants cements the whole reasoning behind their move up the mountain. To teach her son not only to cultivate appreciation for nature but to lean more into their Hawaiian culture, such as language. 'I'm the only person in my family that doesn't speak Hawaiian fluently so it's a really big thing for me now that I have a child. You can lose so much in one generation and I don't want to be the generation that it's lost in.'

Spending time in the garden and listening to the sounds of the wind, the trees and the birds is helping her hear the words of her ancestors. 'As far back as we can go across the world our languages were sounds mimicked from nature,' she says. 'For us, we have seventy-eight words for rain. The colour of the sky when the rain is coming down, the rain when it's light, the rain when it's hard. Little changes are so important and a really big part of the revitalisation of our language. To learn these words so that we can clearly learn to fully love and understand the natural world.'

The biggest piece of advice Wai'ala has for people is to see nature as our mother. 'We call her Mother Earth for a reason. When we think of her as our mother and think about what mothers really do, there is nothing that she won't do to make us better people and to help us.'

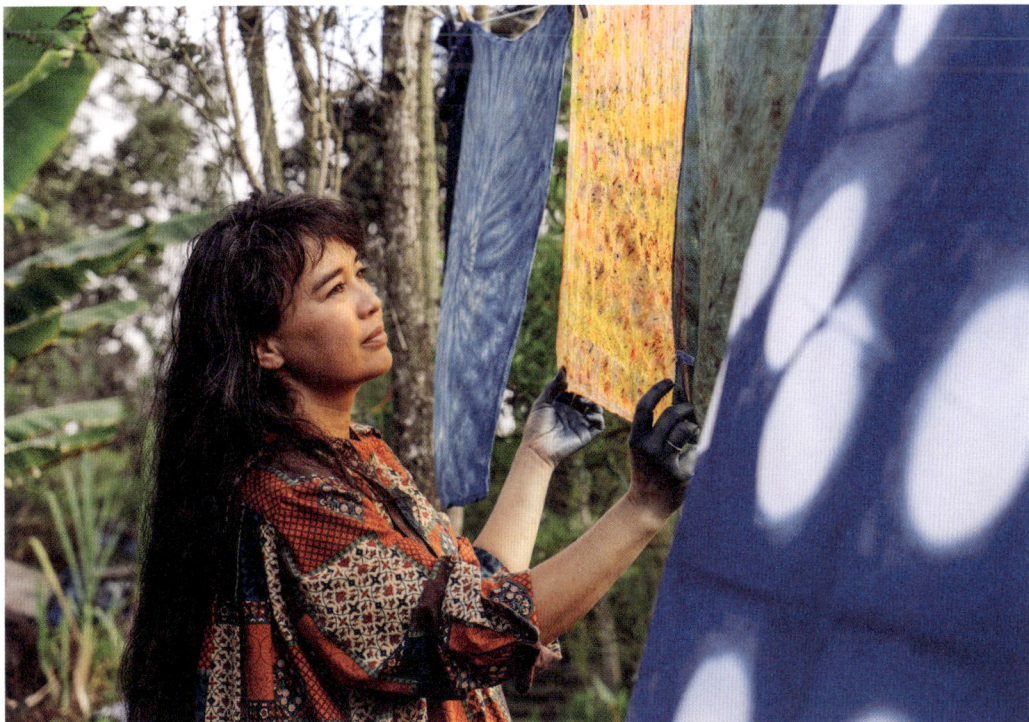

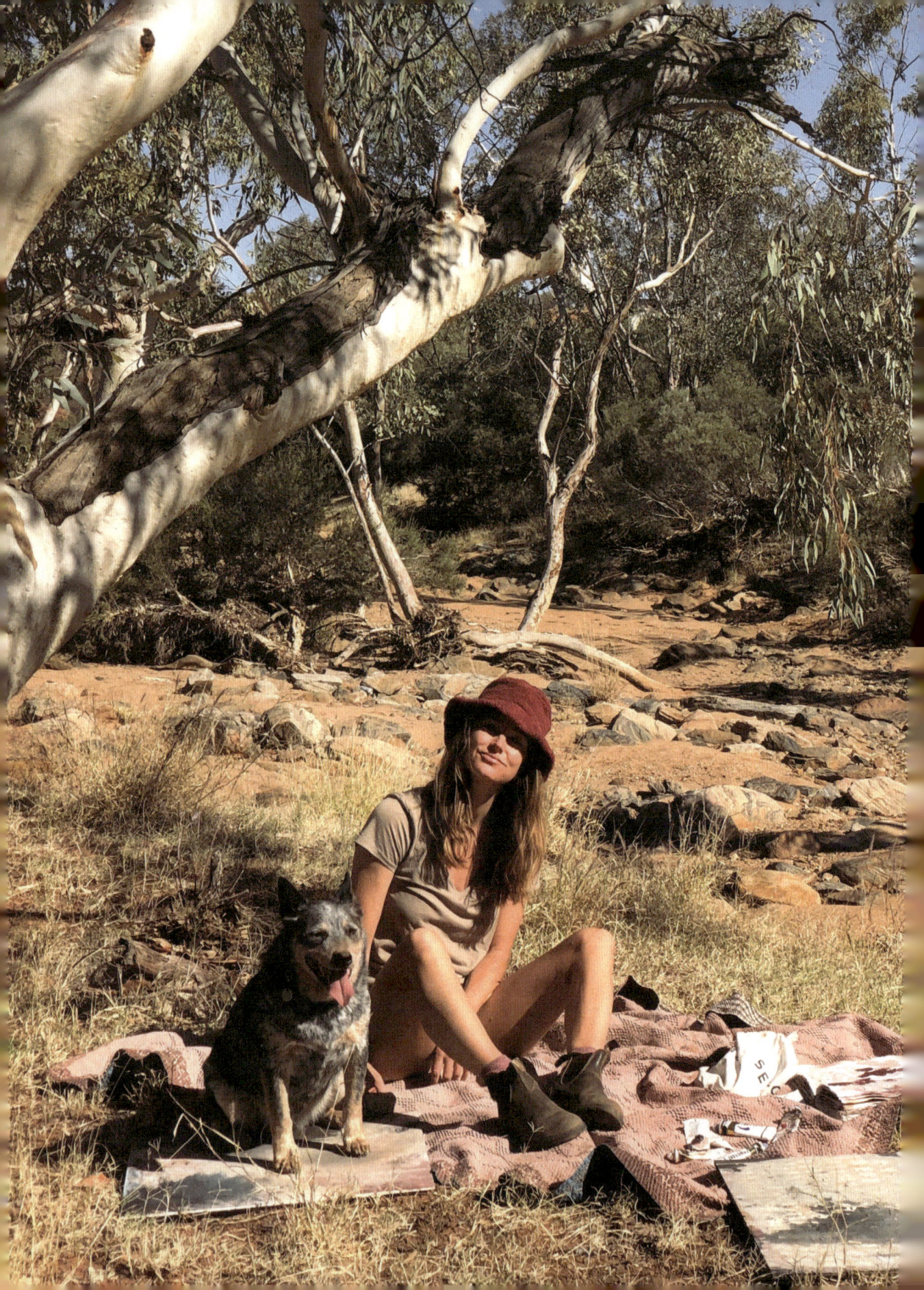

Art

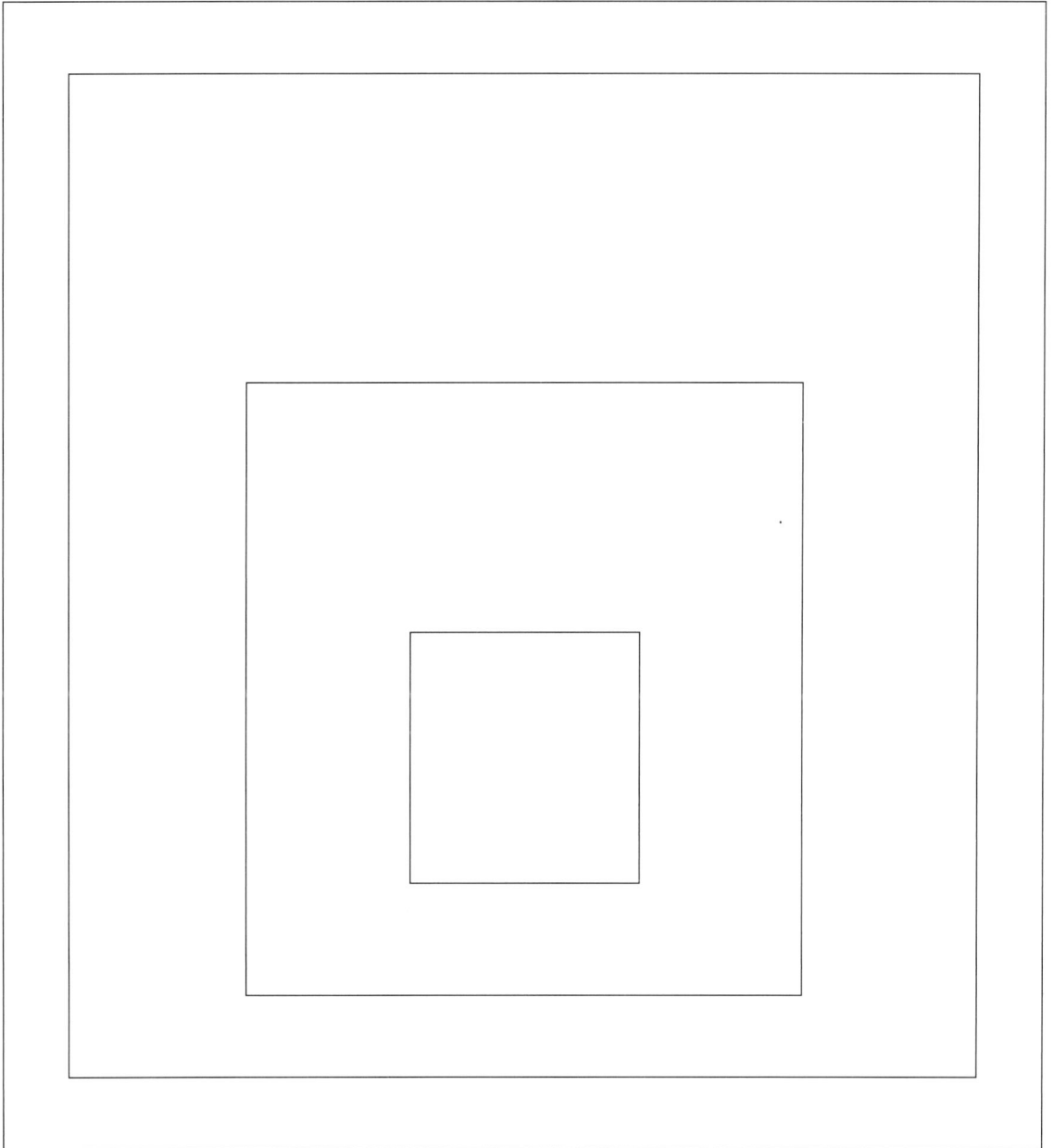

Using found materials and the landscape for creativity

Paige
Northwood

● Australia

Initially setting off with just her tent and some camping equipment, artist Paige Northwood travelled to the centre of Australia to observe the Hermannsburg Potters, a group of Indigenous women creating handmade ceramic pots. Even though she was told the group didn't take volunteers, she stuck around to 'help out' – a visit that ended up lasting three and a half years.

'I used to live in Aboriginal communities and would watch Elders paint. I saw that they were really tapping into something when they were painting. I became interested in how you could stand in front of their work and have physical experiences. I think I absorbed, through my observation of what they were doing, that kind of practice.'

Being raised on the east coast of New South Wales, Australia, Paige always felt a strong connection to the beach. She remembers endless days on the sand watching her dad surf and collecting shells with her mother to make mobiles. This was a practice that not only inspired and influenced her creativity from a young age, but also her connection to nature. Paige believes that our landscape forms part of our identity. 'I didn't know any of the plants when I went to Central Australia, so I felt a little bit alien. There was none of that familiarity or connection but there was the intrigue.'

You can see in Paige's work how her surroundings have influenced her art. Starting out as a ceramic artist, her work has evolved over the years to include paintings allowing her to be more expressive and make bigger work. Paige credits the earth and the rich colours she saw in the outback as the reason why she now predominantly uses pigments and clay that she collects from nature in her work. 'It feels like growing your vegetables. That you're part of the process, a cycle you've been involved in. If I buy commercial clay or acrylic paints, I'm cut off from the source of it all.'

Moving back to the east coast, Paige's work evolved again. 'I'm a little sponge and I absorb everything around me both consciously and unconsciously. In the escarpment behind me there are lots of mosses and I live right next to the ocean, so now all my work is changing to mossy green earth tones and blues.' She believes we form a bond with the things around us.

As a young child of only four years old, Paige remembers experiencing what she would call 'flow state'. 'I have a memory of being so absorbed in what I was doing that time was irrelevant. It was pure presence and the feeling has always stayed with me. As an adult it seems to constantly be an effort to get back to that present inner child.' To invoke this feeling, Paige will meditate for fifteen minutes to an hour before beginning work on any new canvas, a practice that has now become somewhat of a ritual.

It hasn't always been easy as Paige has had to give up a lot to follow this way of life. 'It wasn't until my thirties that I got to know myself and what I needed. I definitely came up against the obstacles of social conditioning and what I thought I was supposed to be doing – to have a career and look a certain way. I did try those things, but they didn't feel right. So I had to let them go and there was a lot of fight around it.' As a practising artist, Paige must have self-belief to confront

The wonder of nature

the exposing nature of exhibiting her work to other people. Art tends to be a solo endeavour, and while she doesn't create for other people, witnessing people connect with her work and the conversations it can start make the pursuit worth it.

Reflecting on her place in the art world, Paige says she feels confident and empowered by her fellow female artists. 'In some ways I'm surrounded by that bubble but I know that's not necessarily representative of what's actually going on. It's hard to stomach, but we are progressing and working towards equality. We're not there yet but there is progress.' This thought mirrors Paige's hope in witnessing the regenerative capabilities of the bush after a fire. 'We all have that potential. Things will regrow and life will come back. Watching things start to shoot out of the ground, you can feel a sense of appreciation for how intelligent nature is,' says Paige with a sense of optimism for the future of women and nature.

'For people who might not see themselves as creative or an artist, there are ways to tap into it. I find that being in nature allows a letting go and an aliveness to happen.'

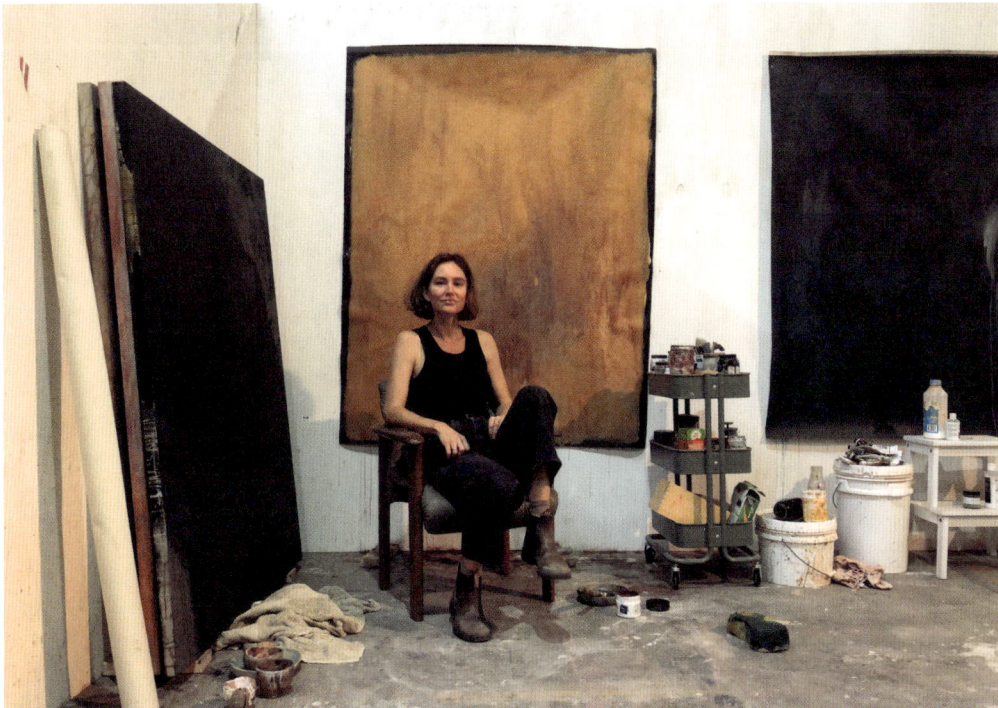

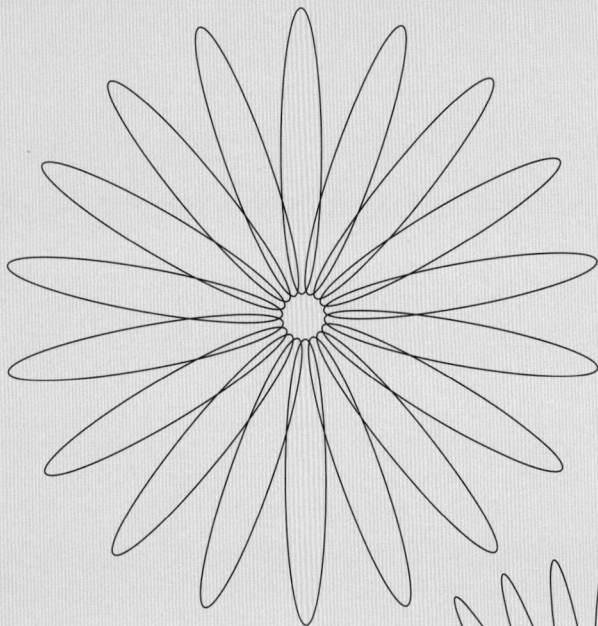

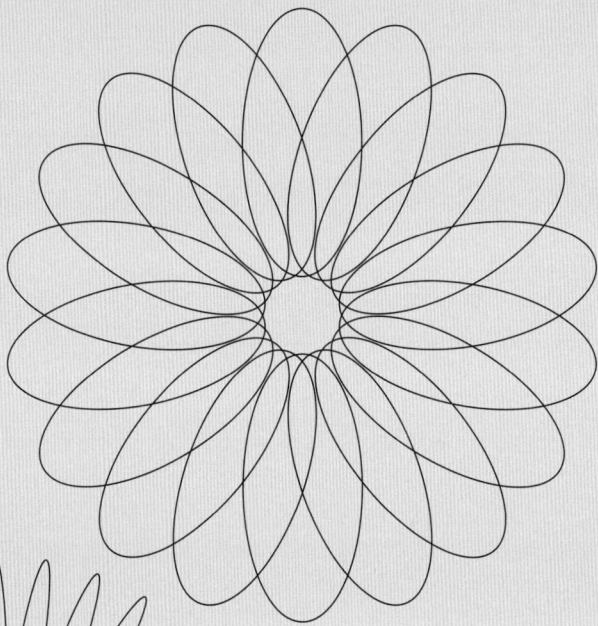

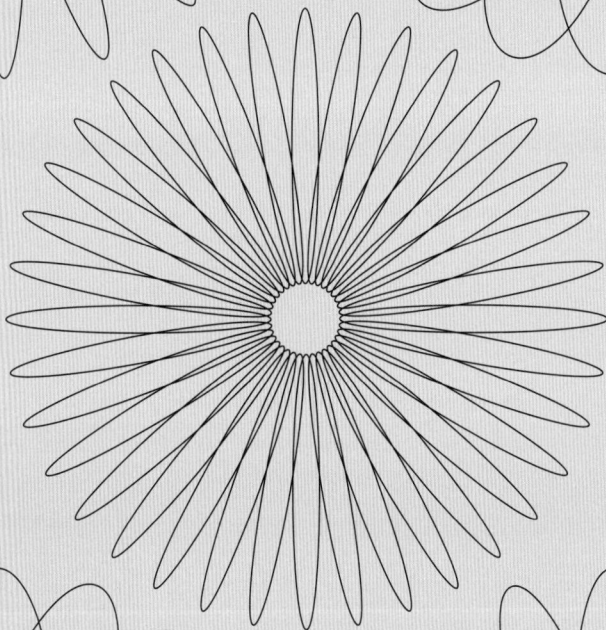

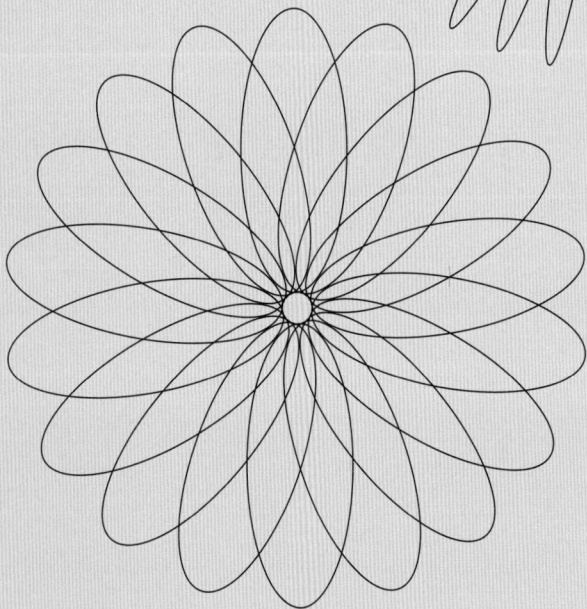

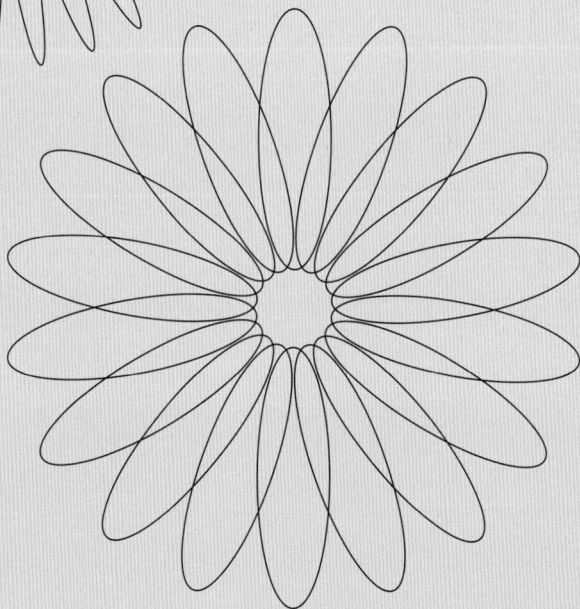

Nature drawing for exploring your creativity

Inspired by Paige Northwood

Creativity is an essential part of life. Many of us would not describe ourselves as creative. Maybe our attempts at portraits come out more like stick figures, but creativity is in each of us. How else would humans have progressed throughout history? Without new ideas and the practice of trial and error, we would not have all of the wonderful progress we currently enjoy.

There are countless TED talks, scientific papers and new professions cropping up supporting the idea that creative expression can improve mental and physical health, such as:

- reducing stress, anxiety and depression by calming nervous system activity
- enabling emotional expression that may be otherwise suppressed
- strengthening neural pathways and improving brain function by learning new skills.

Creating something doesn't always need to have a purpose. Think of children painting or conjuring up characters in a make-believe game. Creativity can spark joy and bring about a sense of playfulness and pleasure. In a time where there is so much worry, uncertainty and fear, making something just for the fun of it might be just the panacea we all need.

Perhaps writing stories, playing the piano or cooking on-the-spot recipes in the kitchen feels overwhelming because it might not turn out the way you expected, but I guarantee not many people created masterpieces on the first try. Nature shows us that perfection is not the prerequisite of beauty. There are no straight lines or matching colours when looking out at the horizon at sunset. By using nature as a muse and allowing imperfections to flourish, creativity can be nurtured.

⟶

To begin ●

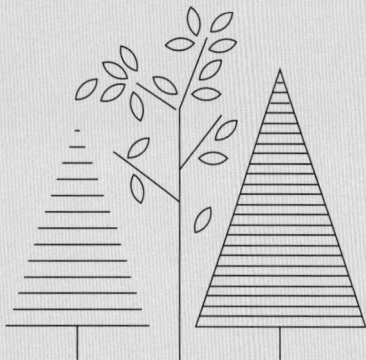

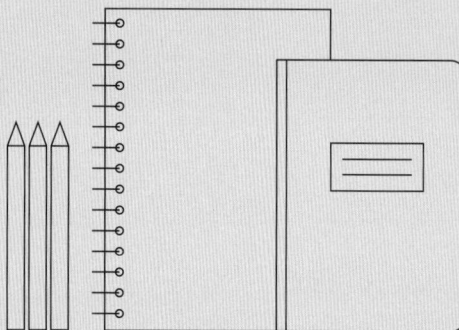

● 1

Go outside somewhere with plants and trees. It could be your garden, the local park or a forest.

● 2

Take with you a small notebook or drawing pad and some pencils.

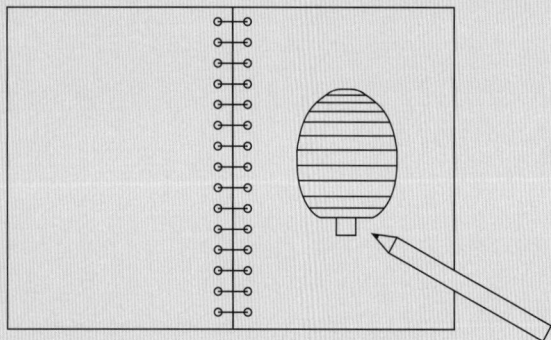

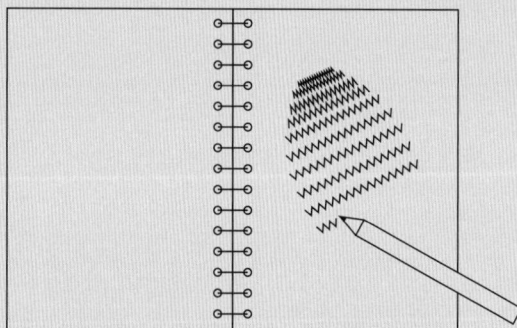

● 6

Once you feel like you have explored enough visually, start to sketch what you see.

● 7

Take your time. You may want to draw from different angles or try shading some areas or using colours.

The wonder of nature

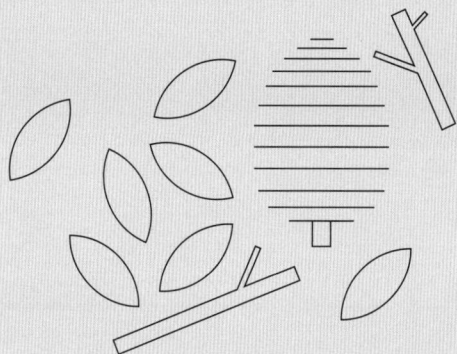

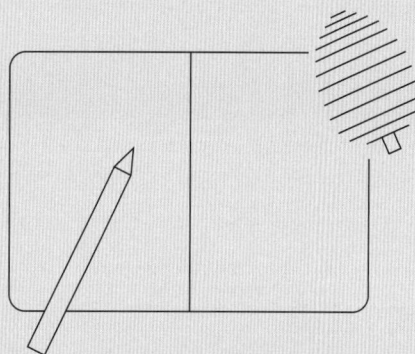

● 3
Look around at fallen leaves, pine cones or flowers until you find something that catches your eye.

● 4
Sit with your natural object and deeply observe the textures, colours and patterns you see.

● 5
You might want to write down some notes so that you can really capture the essence of the object.

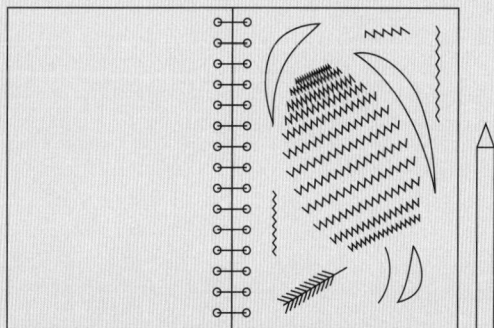

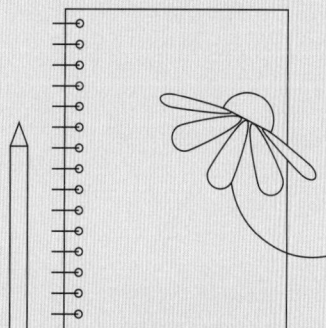

● 8
Don't worry if you think your drawing looks completely different to the real object.

● 9
Once you are finished with your sketches, place the item back where you found it.

● 10
Continue this practice whenever you see something that catches your eye or when you feel like you need a boost in creativity.

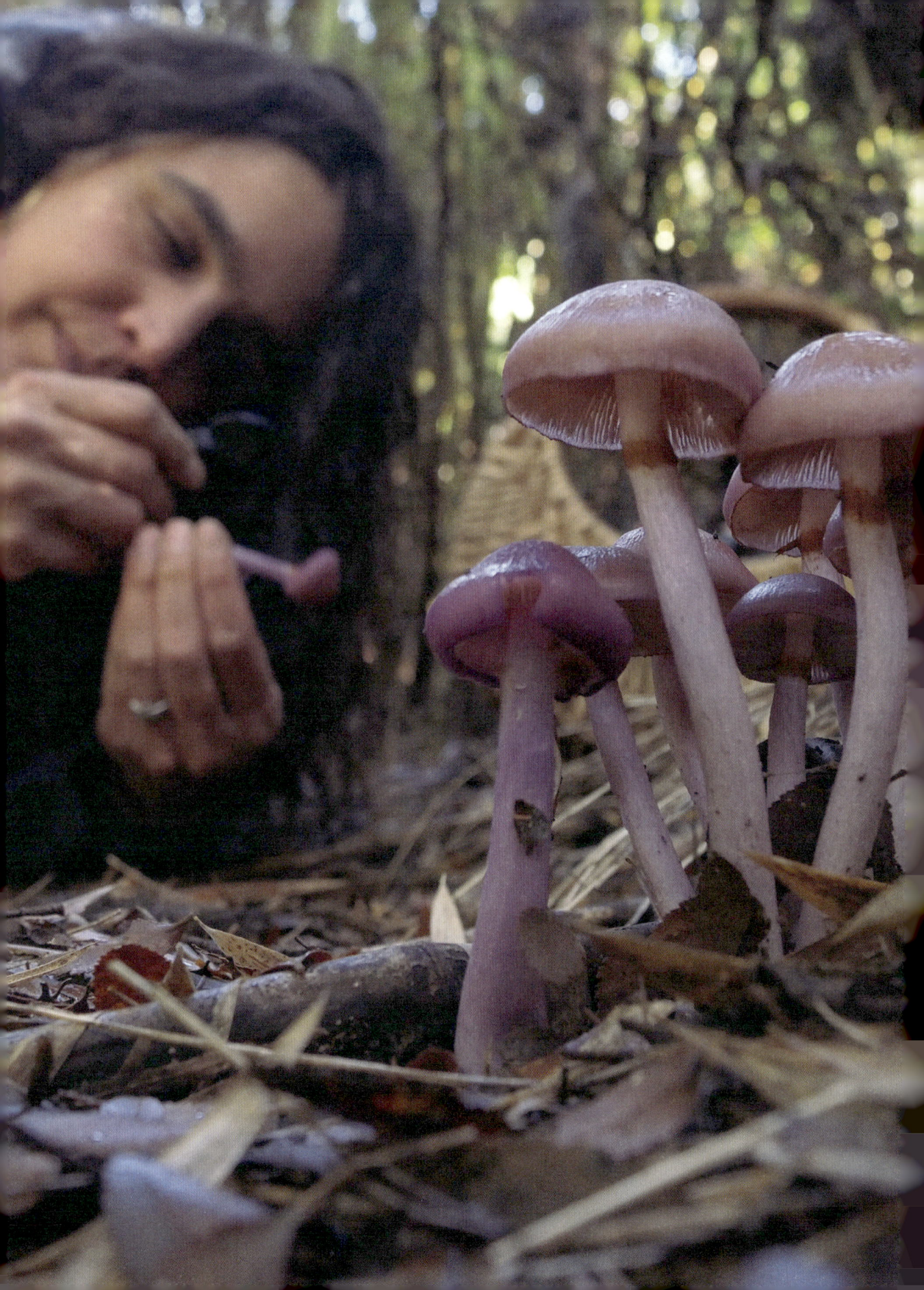

Mycology

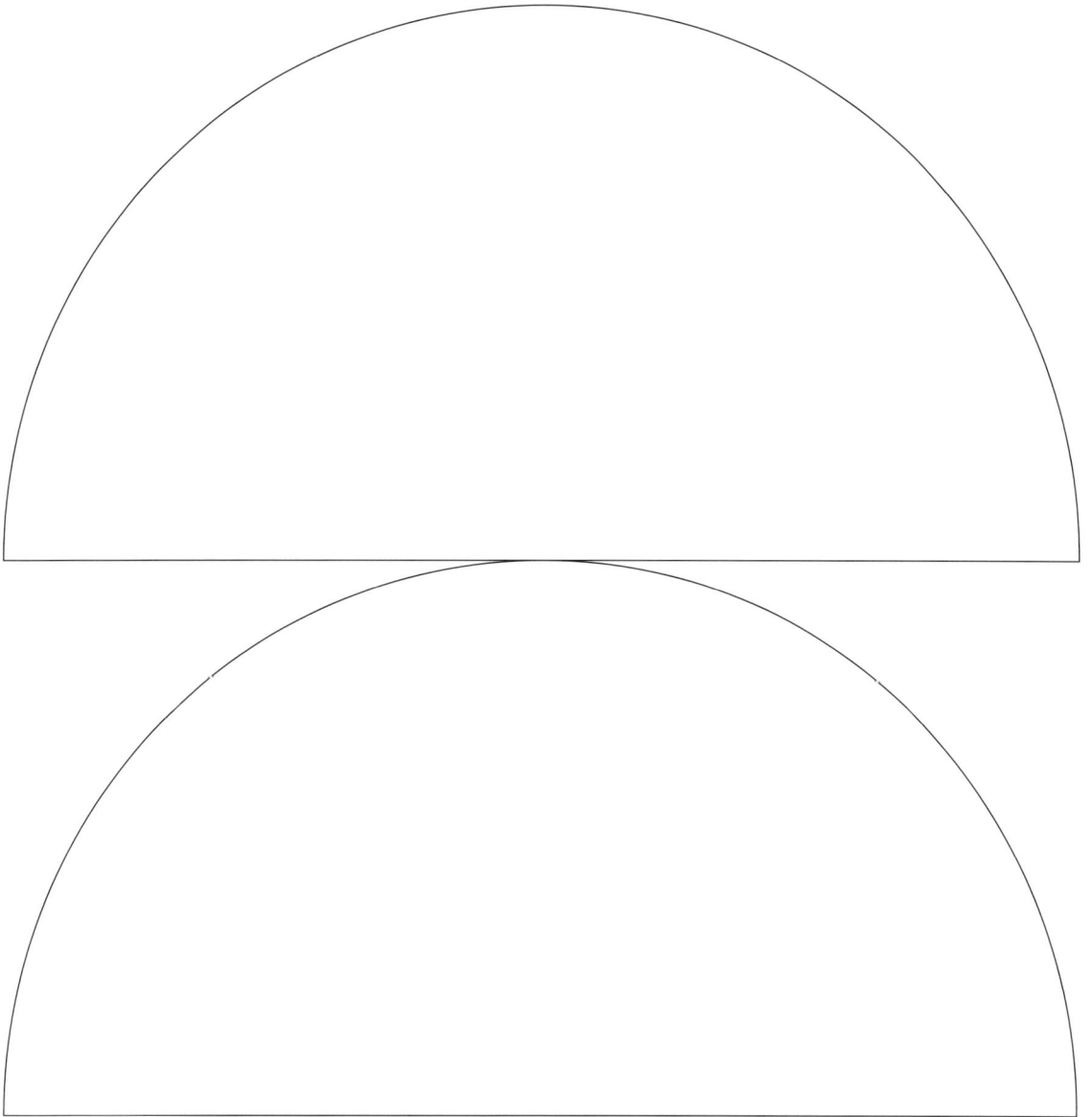

Exploring and highlighting the wonders of fungi

Giuliana Furci

● Chile

Giuliana Furci from Santiago, Chile, formed The Fungi Foundation in response to a lack of educational opportunities in her country. She believed she had only two choices: leave Chile to study abroad or create what was missing. So, she decided to dedicate her life's work to ensure nobody would ever have to leave their country again if they wanted to study mycology (the science of fungi).

The Fungi Foundation was established in Chile in 2012 and offered education in mycology. Since then, the organisation has gone on to design and launch a global mycological curriculum alongside research and conservation efforts. 'Chile is currently the only country in the world that includes fungi in their environmental impact assessments on equal footing to plants and animals. A lot of this is a result of our direct work,' she says proudly. Giuliana and her team have also been working on mapping the world's underground mycorrhizal networks and pushing for mycological inclusive language to be included in conservation and biodiversity frameworks.

But what does all of this mean? Fungi, as Giuliana explains, are their own kingdom. They are not animals, plants or minerals but their own grouping of organic organisms. 'When we say fungi, it's like saying animals. An oyster mushroom and a truffle are both fungi but they are as closely related as a worm and an elephant.' The diversity in the fungi kingdom is immense and they are found in all ecosystems. 'They are ubiquitous; they live in freshwater, sea water and at altitude. They live wherever there is organic matter really.'

Thanks to the work of Giuliana, as well as mainstream documentary films and multiple books being released on the fungi kingdom, popularity is rising for this once under-acknowledged part of nature. With popularity comes funding for research, and over recent years some breathtaking discoveries have been made. Examples such as certain fungi's ability to clean up toxic waste, decompose plastics and even convert radiation into energy are reported on The Fungi Foundation's website. Further peer-reviewed scientific studies are also currently being undertaken thanks to Giuliana's hard work.

Giuliana says that the fungi chose her and she did not purposely set out to work in this space. 'I had an encounter with a fungus and something sparked. I tried to do other things and I just couldn't,' she says. From an early age, Giuliana knew that she wanted to give back, initially setting out to study social work before moving onto landscaping and ecology. It wasn't until she was studying seaweeds and algae that she first encountered the world of fungi and her path was finally found.

In the world of mycology, women are thriving. 'There are many women working in labs all around the world. Mexico has many incredible female mycologists as well as Brazil and the United Kingdom,' she says. For Giuliana personally, there were times where she was questioned on who was looking after her son when out in the field and feeling like she was just filling a gender quota but all in all, she found the mycological world safe and inviting. 'It's not an impediment being a woman in this field in my experience.'

Over the years there are two profound lessons that Giuliana has been pondering thanks to this work. 'One is that fungi demonstrates that individuals don't exist; that no one exists without others,' she says in relation to the interconnectedness of fungal networks under our soil and their role in helping plants and animals to thrive. 'And secondly, they demonstrate that the end of one life form isn't the end of life. Death isn't an end.' A reference to how fungi break down all the living matter on Earth.

From the creation of medicines to some of our favourite foods, supplying us with sturdy materials, to breaking down our waste, fungi form an essential part of our existence on the planet. Giuliana encourages all of us to learn and appreciate what fungi already do for us, rather than looking at them as completely separate organisms.

'Most women like having a glass of wine or beer, a chocolate or a coffee. None of that would exist without fungi because the yeasts that make all of those are fungi.'

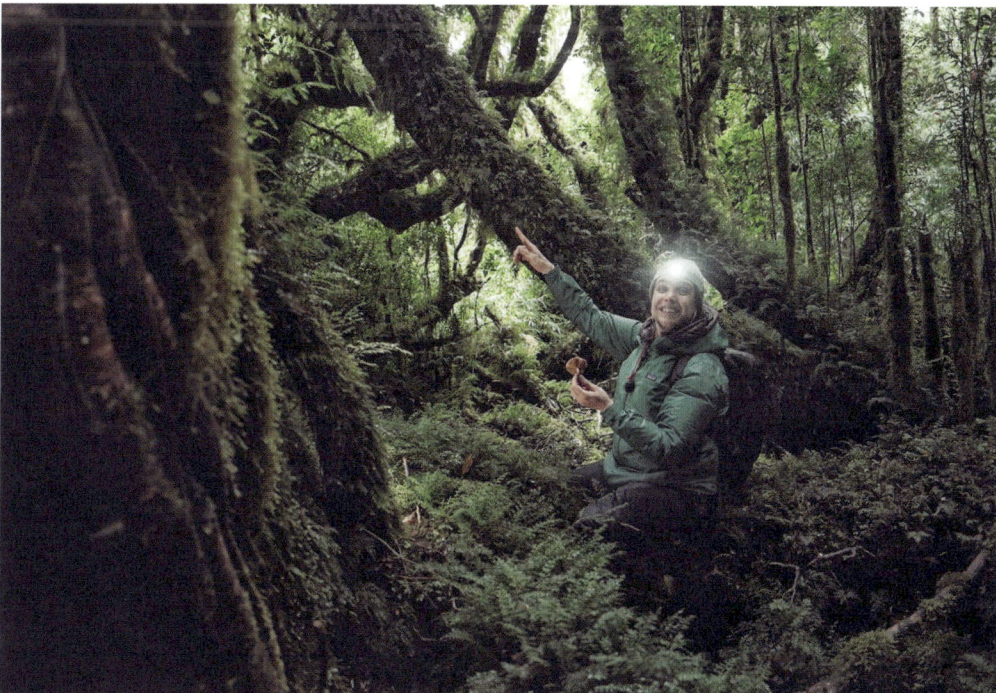

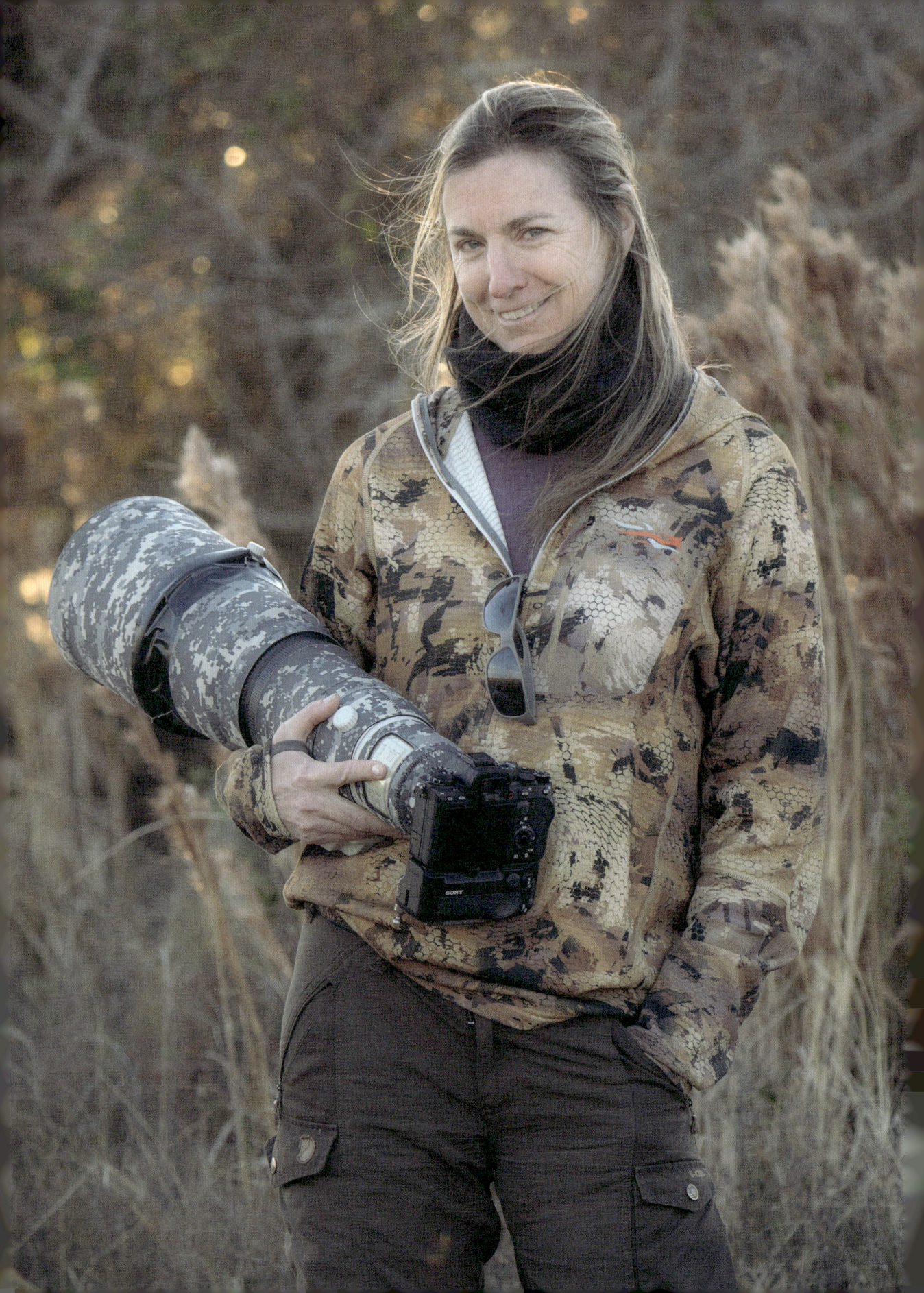

Wildlife photography

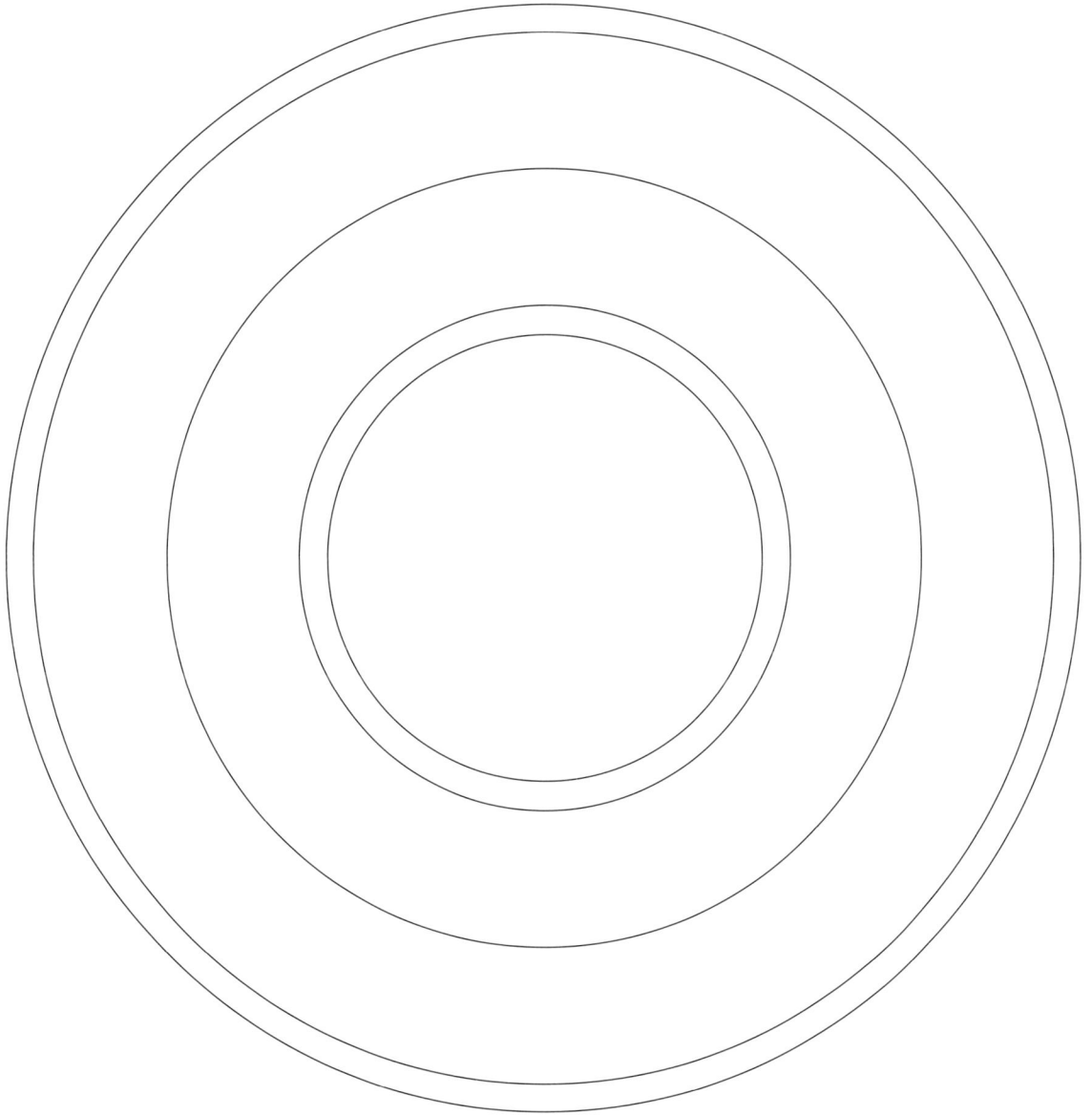

Capturing images for education and conservation

Melissa Groo

● USA

With experience in education and teaching, Melissa Groo credits spending two field seasons in Africa observing and recording data on wild elephants for building the skills she now utilises in her career as a wildlife photographer. 'It was there that I really began to understand how to frame a scene and composition. I wasn't a photographer then, but my mentor, Katy Payne, knew I had a sense for being able to anticipate interesting behaviour and stories unfolding.'

Growing up in Manhattan, USA, Melissa wasn't exposed to a lot of nature in her youth, a seemingly unlikely beginning for a woman who would go on to be featured in some of the most well-known wildlife magazines and win multiple awards for her images of wild animals. As a child she adored her cats and dogs and rescuing insects from the pool at her family's home. 'I thought I would be a vet when I grew up, but I couldn't stand the sight of blood, so I knew that was out. I always had this strong empathy, almost to a fault, for animals and their welfare.'

In the late 1990s Melissa took a trip with her father to sea kayak in Alaska where she was fortunate enough to encounter a humpback whale fluking. 'It raised its tail up out of the water as it came up and I was just totally smitten by that. I went back to Ohio where I was living at the time and read everything I could about whales,' she recounts this time as a great inspiration for her. This is when she came upon the work of Katy, who at the time was at the forefront of research into whale sounds. Melissa boldly went up to her after a seminar and expressed her love of whales, a conversation which carried on into a lunch and eventually a job offer to join Katy's research team at Cornell University and subsequent trips to Africa.

After five years working with Katy, Melissa took a break from research to become a mother. It wasn't until her daughter was in day care that she decided to try photography. After a couple of years playing around with macro and landscape styles, she discovered bird and wildlife photography. 'That was it for me. I finally felt like I had found my thing. It was like a great marriage of my love for animals and an artistic aesthetic sense that I never really had an outlet for,' she says. Learning everything she could about the best equipment, light and composition, Melissa then focused her attention on studying natural history to perfect her craft. 'I really knew how important it was to understand animal behaviour. First to know where to find them and secondly to understand the signs and clues that there is about to be a story.'

Melissa most enjoys photographing the 'underdogs' – animals that are often not well understood or commonly persecuted – such as foxes, bobcats and coyotes. 'People regard them as varmints, not understanding they have a really important role to play in the ecosystem with rodent control, acting as scavengers and cleaning up carcasses. There are so many important reasons that we need predators. I'm always trying to awaken people to the necessity of these animals and to the fact that they have feelings and families.' When questioned about her favourite photo, Melissa mentions a beautiful image of a bobcat mother sitting in the snow with her kit nuzzling into her, a show of affection very rarely captured by such an elusive and misunderstood animal.

What started out as a creative hobby has now turned into the pursuit of conservation and protection of wild animals and their habitats. Melissa takes photographs and writes articles because she believes this should be important for all of us, 'Our fate is inextricably linked to the fate of so many wild creatures. What befalls them, befalls us.'

Talking on her most profound lessons from nature, Melissa notes patience as one of her biggest takeaways from wildlife photography. 'I grew up in New York City and I'm used to living a fast-paced life. Sitting and watching elephants at a glacial pace and just being attuned to every movement, waiting and watching taught me patience, which has been completely vital as a wildlife photographer.'

'Wild animals treasure their families and feel love, joy and fear. I really want to invoke empathy, understanding and appreciation and to get people to care for something they don't have any experience with.'

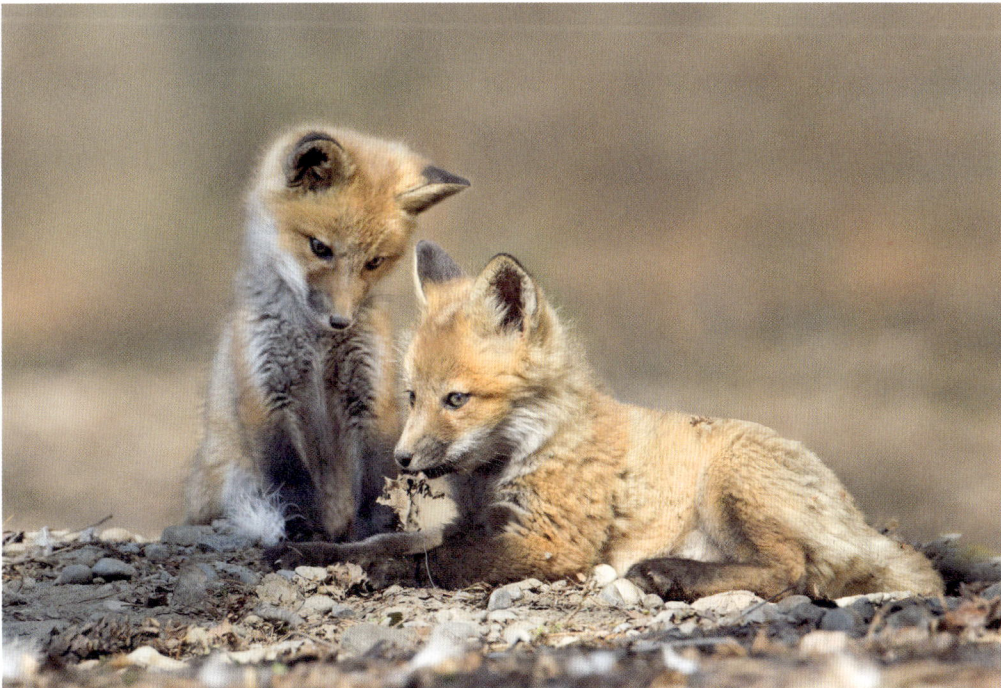

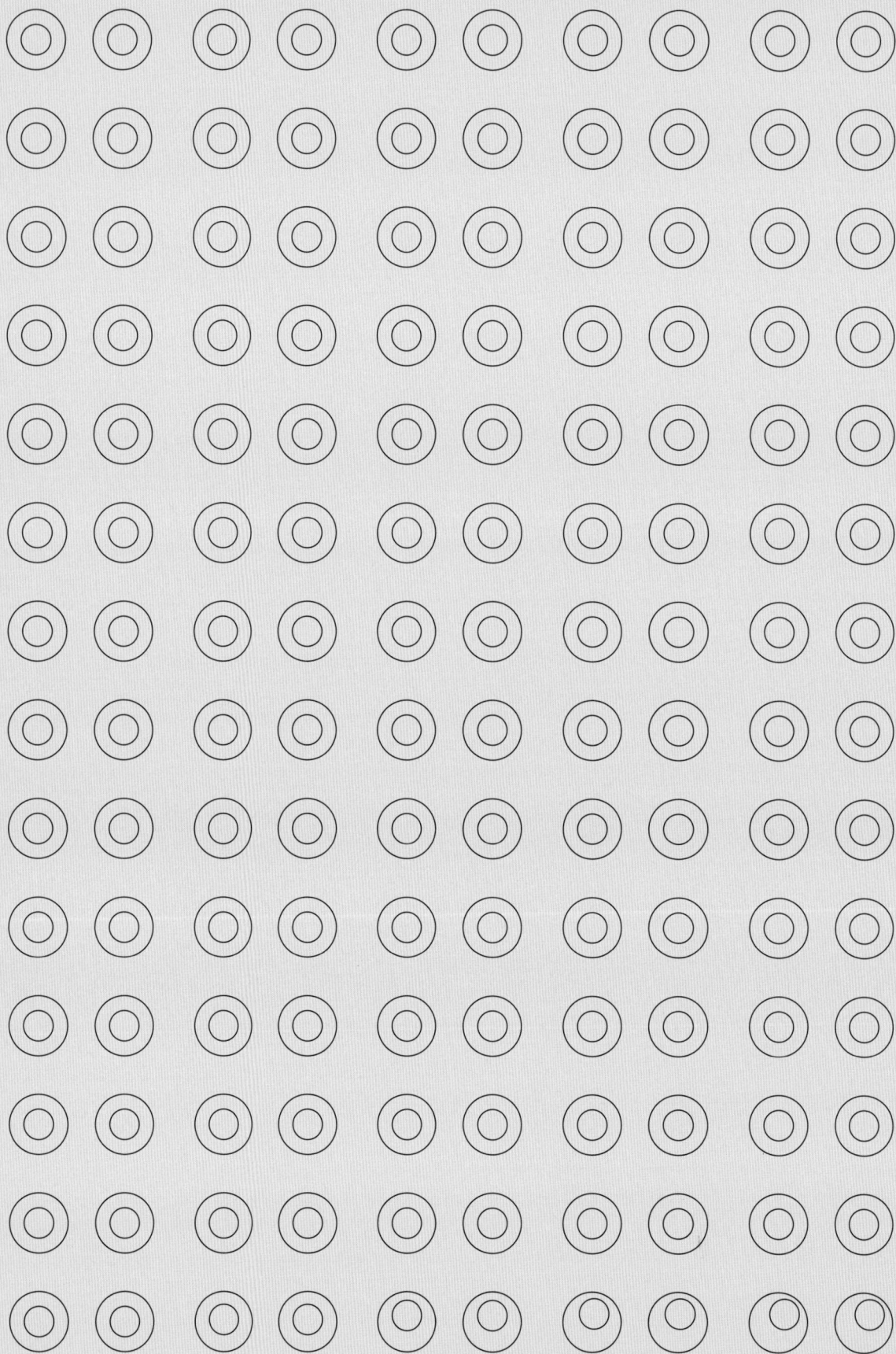

Animal observation for slowing down and cultivating patience

Inspired by Melissa Groo

There is a particular type of wonder we can experience when in the presence of animals. In recent years, research has labelled this 'wildlife-inspired awe'. It is the feeling of emotions and strong connection to a particular moment signified by wild animals. I remember driving through a national park in Sri Lanka and seeing a herd of elephants. We pulled over and watched them for a while before I saw a little calf weaving between the legs of its mother. In that very moment, time stood still and I felt such a reverence for these animals that my eyes began to well up. I now know this was 'wildlife-inspired awe'.

Animals have been inextricably linked to human existence and development throughout history. Without oxen we would not have had the ability to move large materials. Without horses we couldn't have travelled long distances over land. Without bees we would not have pollinated plants for our fruits and vegetables. And, essentially, humans are also part of the animal kingdom. By observing animals in their natural environment, we can begin to learn a little more about our original temperament and behaviour before the cars, phones and fluorescent lights arrived. Other benefits can include:

- decreased feelings of loneliness and isolation
- increased compassion for other species
- reduced blood pressure and cortisol (stress hormone)
- better focus and patience
- improved immune strength when having pets in the household or spending time outdoors.

The practice of animal observation involves mindfully watching and listening to (maybe smelling but probably not touching) animals. Think of bird watching, a hobby that has been practised since the late 1800s, whereby the 'birder' will intentionally go to a place for the purpose of observing birds. This can be for recreation or for gathering research but both involves sitting still for long stints of time and just witnessing the behaviour of birds. In a time when many of us are seeking more mindful experiences as well as more time in nature, the practice of animal observation can facilitate both of these needs.

$\longrightarrow$

To begin ●

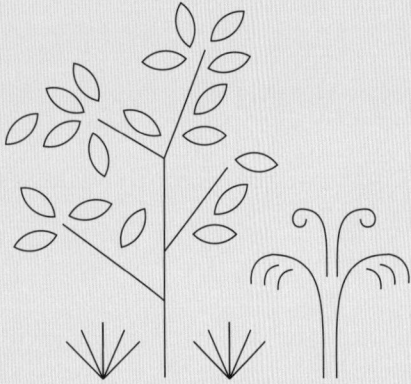

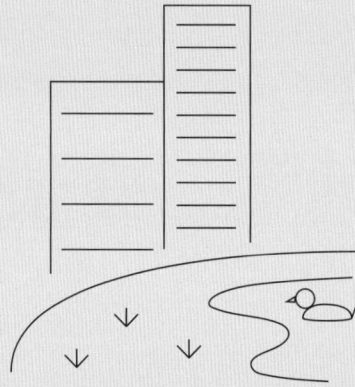

● 1
Choose a place where you believe you will be able to safely sit for an amount of time and where you are likely able to see animals.

● 2
Don't worry if you live in a city, the animals you observe don't have to be exotic lions, monkeys or kangaroos, simply watching an insect or a pigeon can be just as effective. It is also possible to do this practice with pets.

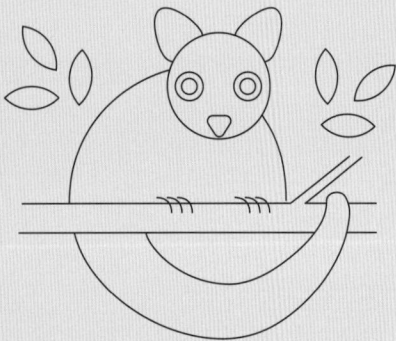

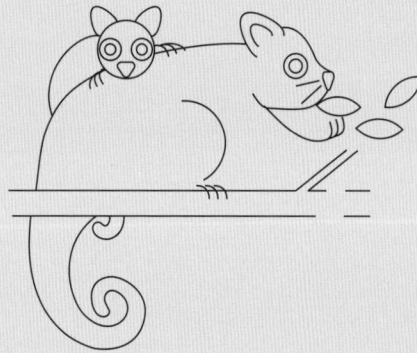

● 5
Focus on the animal you have chosen and simply observe what they are doing. Can you see them interacting with other animals? Are they making any sounds? Are they building something, eating something or grooming themselves? Do they have babies? What story is this animal telling you?

● 6
Try to pay attention to the behaviour of your chosen animal for at least five minutes or until they leave.

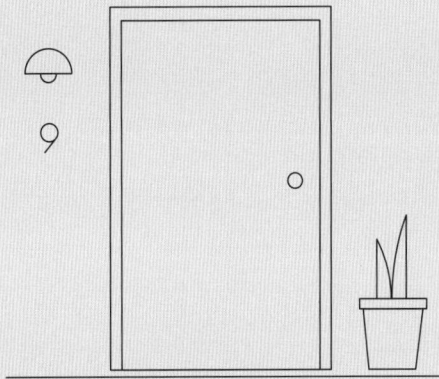

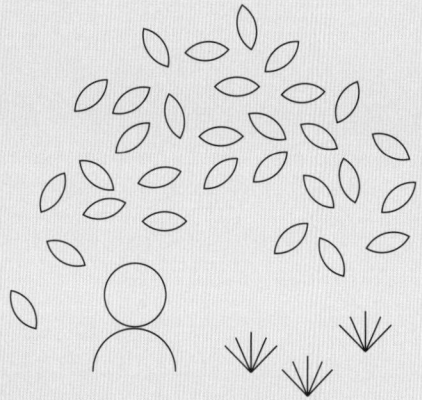

3
Try to leave your phone at home and
dedicate this time to mindfully observing
the animal.

4
It may be easier for you to do this
somewhere away from noise and people
to reduce distractions.

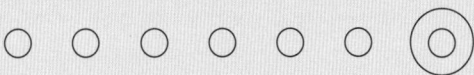

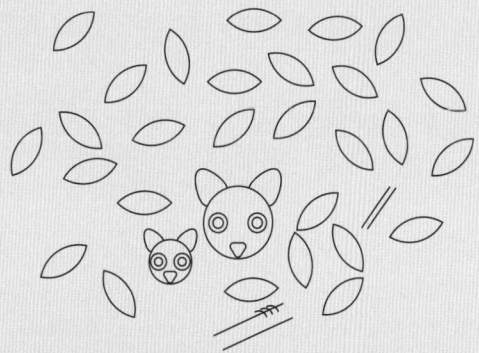

7
Spend some time reflecting after your
observation. Think about how you felt
before the observation and how you feel
now. Have you noticed a difference?

8
If you can, return to this same place
the next day and see if you can find the
same animal. By doing this repeatedly
you can form a relationship with this
animal and your empathy for all animals
is likely to grow.

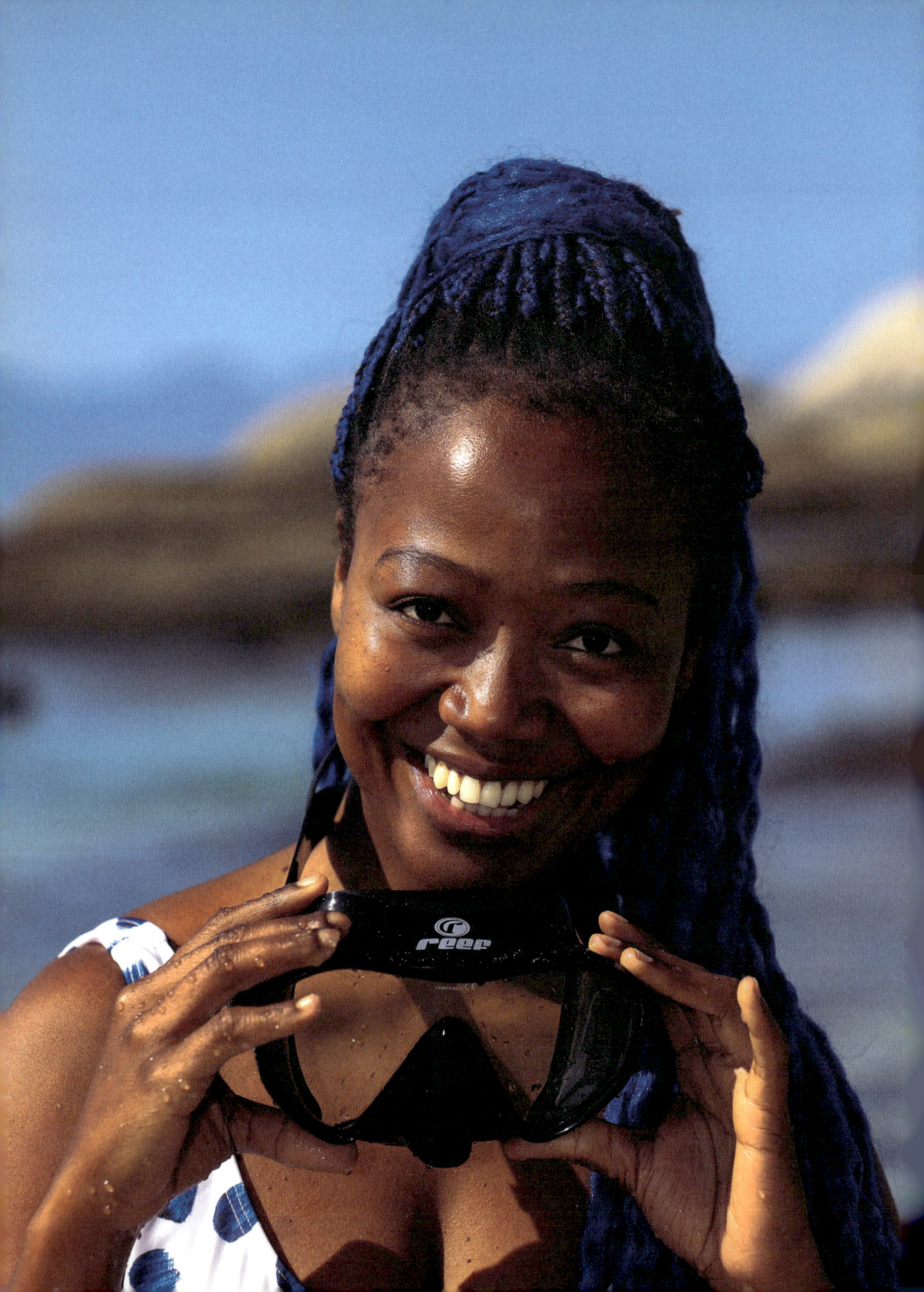

Free diving

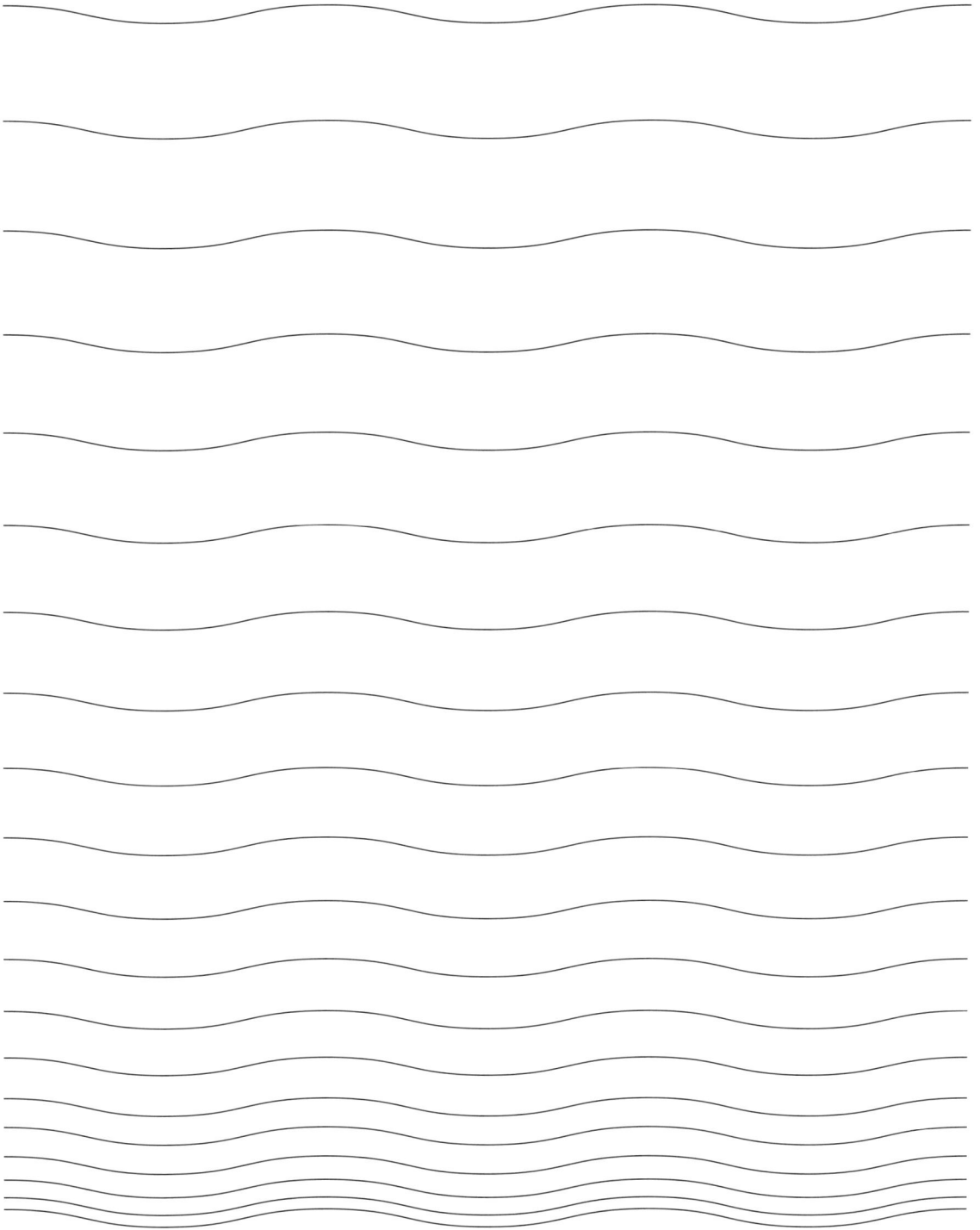

Embracing and encouraging diversity in the ocean

Zandi Ndhlovu

● South Africa

Four minutes and fifteen seconds: that's how long Zandi Ndhlovu of Cape Town, South Africa can hold her breath underwater. She modestly explains that this is only her static breath hold when she is not moving and that if she is expending energy by diving or using camera equipment, it is less. However, it is still hugely impressive and even more so because Zandi grew up a six-hour drive away from the coast and never spent any time in the ocean.

Following the divorce from her husband, Zandi took a trip to Gili Trawangan, Indonesia, where she spontaneously joined a snorkelling trip. 'The further and further we went out there was just this fear. What if something happens out there? Who is going to tell my family?' she recalls of the thoughts she had running through her mind. After having what she describes as a dramatic full-on freak out when she jumped off the boat, Zandi eventually calmed down and went under water. 'That was my first time seeing beneath the surface of the ocean. I was twenty-eight years old and it was the most surreal experience of my life.'

'When you're underwater, you realise that everything looks all kinds of different but it's also the most normal thing. No one looks over at a triggerfish and says, "Why is your head so big?" Everything in the ocean is just what it is. It coexists so beautifully.'

Something Zandi identifies as contributing to her fear of that first snorkelling trip was the fact that there was no one else on that boat who looked like her. 'Sometimes you just need another black person to wink at you and say everything is okay,' she says. This has been a huge driver for her work with creating greater representation in the ocean being Zandi's underlying mission. 'When you think of all the global faces that you can imagine, what would it mean to have that actual representation show up across the world in a way that allows people to identify with the ocean.'

Upon returning home from Indonesia, Zandi continued spending time in the ocean and a few years later she became a certified free-diving instructor. It was during these years of learning that Zandi truly noticed the challenges and lack of diversity within ocean activities in her country. 'Firstly, there is the financial barrier to get your certifications and tally up the dives that grow your competence in the ocean,' she says. 'Secondly, the reminders that I am the one that is different, the one that doesn't belong. That was my greatest challenge.' Zandi says that on almost every dive trip someone would bring up her long-braided hair. 'They would say, "Are you going to dive with all of that hair?" I used to laugh it off but eventually I thought, you don't ask anybody else that question.'

Following this, Zandi created The Black Mermaid Foundation to encourage more people of colour into the ocean. A documentary film, a YouTube channel and multiple partnerships later, The Black Mermaid brand and message has grown. 'When I started this journey, I was probably one of the most vocal voices not just in South Africa but internationally. Now you can see there are more voices in the space. That's important but we definitely still have work to do,' she says.

The wonder of nature

Zandi says that one of the most amazing things she has witnessed in the ocean is a humpback whale and her calf. 'The baby was right on top of the mum, still learning to work its tail. It's one of the most mind-blowing sights underwater,' she says. Hearing the songs of whales makes her feel less alone in the depths. 'It's probably one of the most surreal experiences, especially if you are on a free dive because you're in a world where you're normally by yourself but it feels like the whales come and go with you to the bottom of the ocean and back.'

If you have a glimmer of interest in the ocean, Zandi tells you to just go for it. She recalls looking out at the ocean from a distance while on a mountain bike trail and feeling an unexplained pull. At that time she hadn't yet gone on her trip to Indonesia but something stirred within her. This is what eventually took her down a path away from her corporate job and her comfortable life to a place she could never have dreamed of. 'Allow your heart to lead. When you're afraid and there's a whole lot of uncertainty, that's just the reminder that you're standing on gold.'

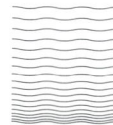

'The ocean has taught me the value of truth as a free diver, because if you cannot be truthful with yourself on a free dive, you put your life in danger. There is no room for ego.'

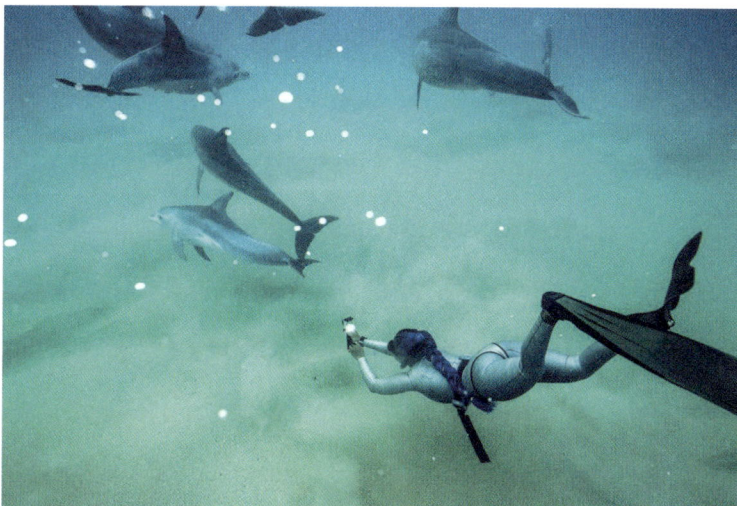

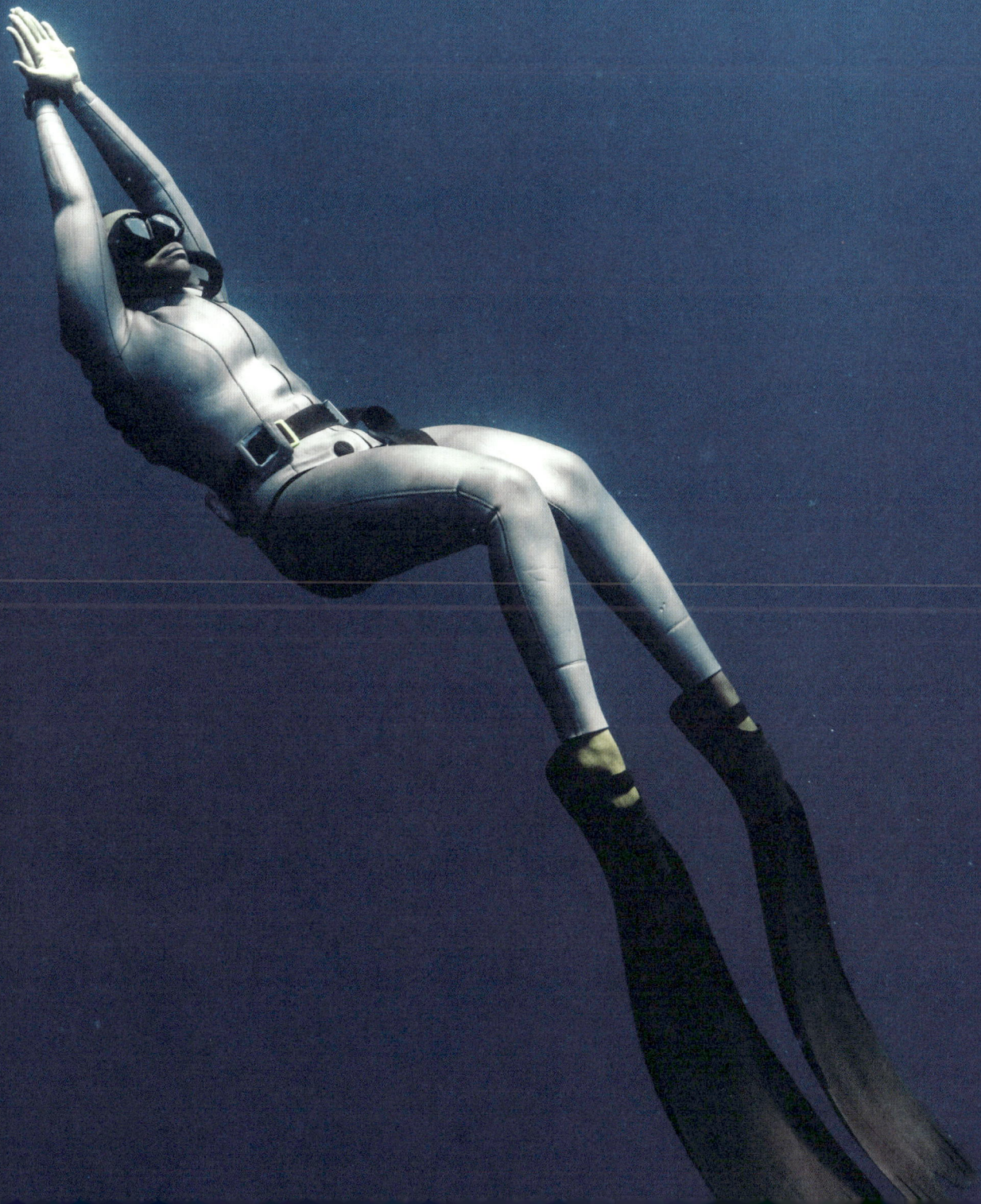

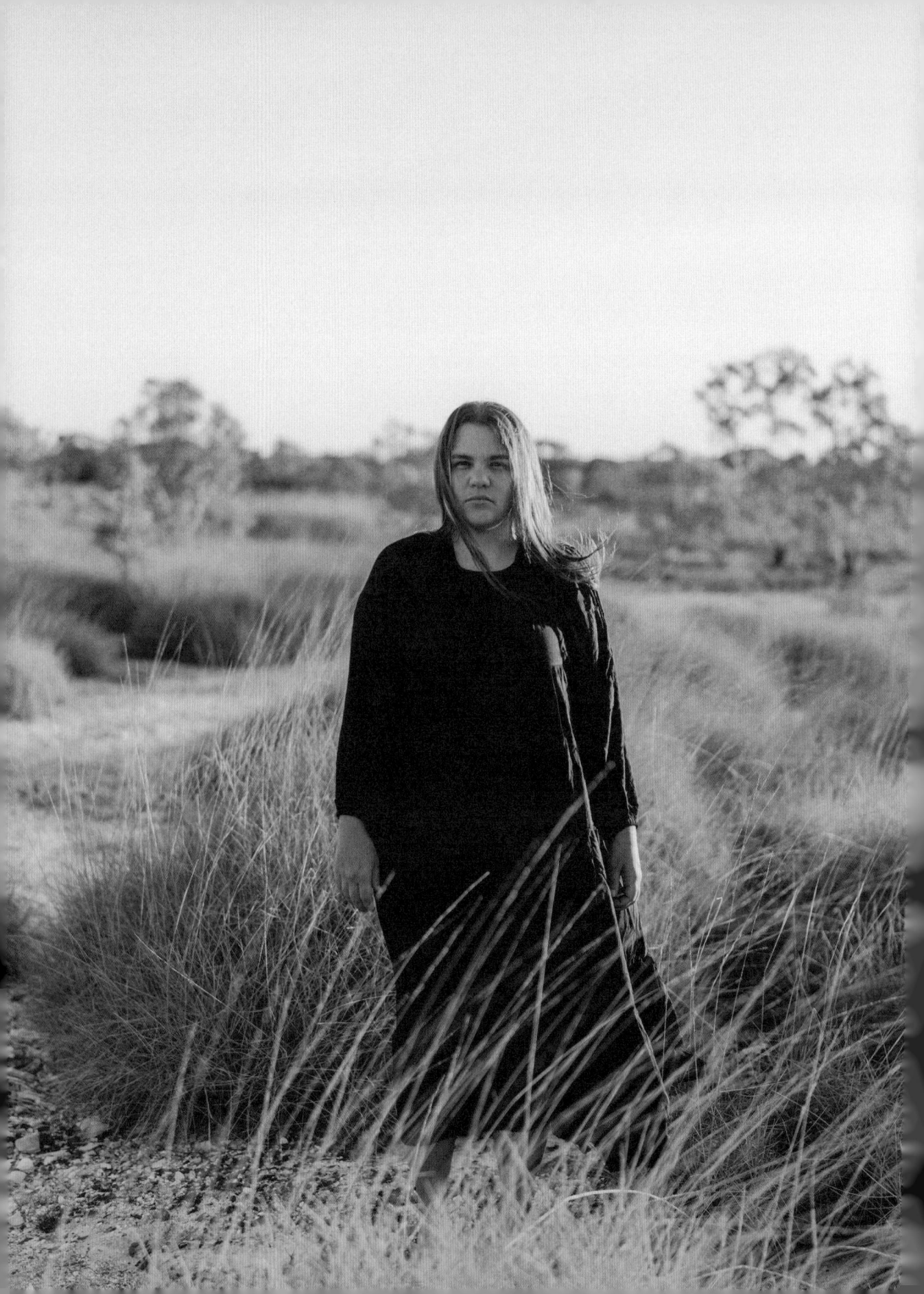

Art and design

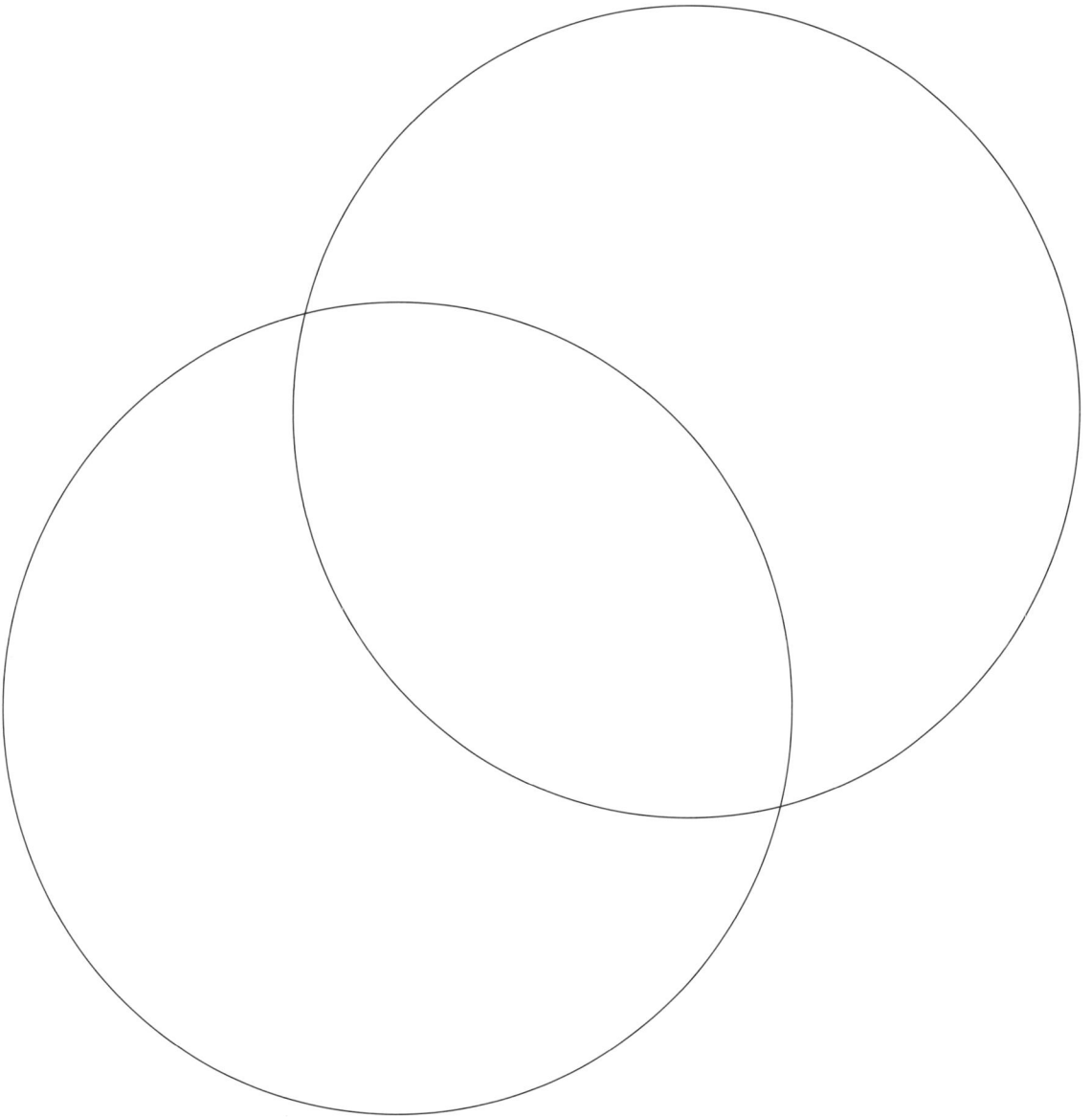

Painting Country to strengthen relationships

Glenda McCulloch

● Australia

What initially started out as Glenda McCulloch experimenting with painting and wanting to showcase her work through social media, quickly grew into four sisters producing art that was in such high demand it was constantly selling out. Now it is rare to see a piece of their art up for sale for long, as they mainly work on private commissions through their business, Cungelella Art. But the sisters don't have fancy studios or expensive equipment, they are simply spending time with each other and creating from what they know and love. 'We don't see it as work. For us, we are just going over to each other's house and having a cup of tea and making some art,' says Glenda describing what has become a very successful business for her and her sisters.

Glenda's Country is Kalkatungu (Kalkadoon), approximately 200 kilometres east from the Northern Territory border in Queensland, Australia. Located on dry desert land, it's not hard to see how the natural earthy tones of the sisters' work has been influenced by what they see. 'We get a lot of our inspiration from Country. Out here, we have this beautiful red dirt and the creamy colours of the stone and in about ninety per cent of our work you will see spinifex grass,' says Glenda. The intimate relationship the sisters have with the landscape means that nature's subtle changes are not lost on them. 'At a certain time of year little purple flowers come out and we'll paint those and the animal tracks that we see. We are lucky because we get to be around our inspiration every day.'

Growing up as one of nine children, six of whom are women, Glenda has fond memories of always being together in what she calls chaos. She remembers their holidays together when they would all go out bush and camp in swags. 'Our dad would catch kangaroo for us to eat around the fire and he would show us Aboriginal artifacts and rocks.' A tradition that he is carrying on with the fourteen grandchildren he has from Glenda and her siblings. 'He will take the kids and show them how to make didgeridoos out of trees and he knows places where they can see stone axe heads,' says Glenda fondly about their connection to the land and people.

As an Aboriginal woman, Glenda knows that her love of the land is part of her culture. 'Blackfellas respect nature. We rely on waterholes and we rely on the land. Protecting the land is more important than money.' For her, it is simple: 'If we don't look after the place we are living on, where are we going to live? We can't just go and live on another planet.'

That ethos is carried over into a second project the sisters have started, a fashion label called Myrrdah. Using only Australian materials and manufacturers, they create artworks that are then printed onto linen and cotton. 'For us, rather than getting it mass-produced with cheap materials, we wanted it to still be a piece of art,' she says. Creating this label was a way for everyone in the family to be involved. The four sisters create the artwork and other siblings and family members help with the production. Family is the epicentre of their work.

Learning to paint and create was not through formal education or lessons. 'Our dad and mum and aunties all painted when we were growing up,' Glenda says. Having that as a normal part of her upbringing is likely what gave her the courage to begin Cungelella Art in 2019. It is also a legacy she hopes to pass on to her children as they grow up surrounded by creative women and family who love nature. 'Aboriginal people want to look after Country and our people.'

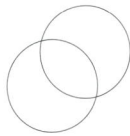

'Blackfellas respect nature. We rely on waterholes and we rely on the land. Protecting the land is more important than money. If we don't look after the place we are living on, where are we going to live? We can't just go and live on another planet.'

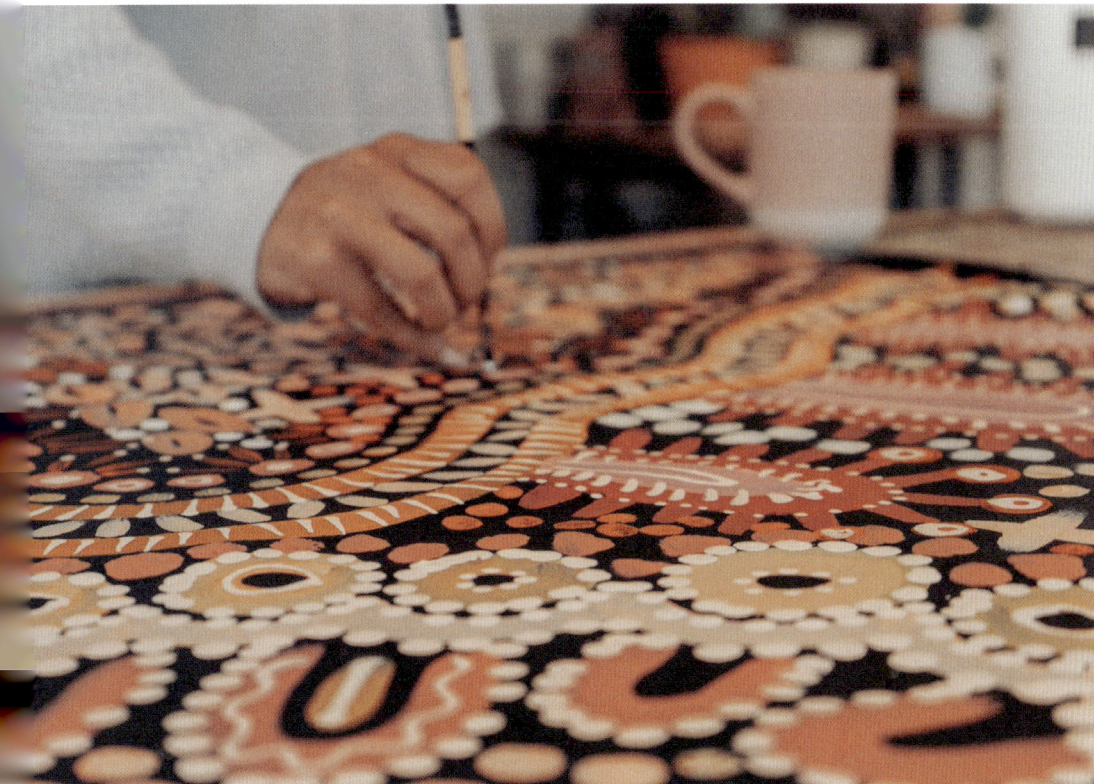

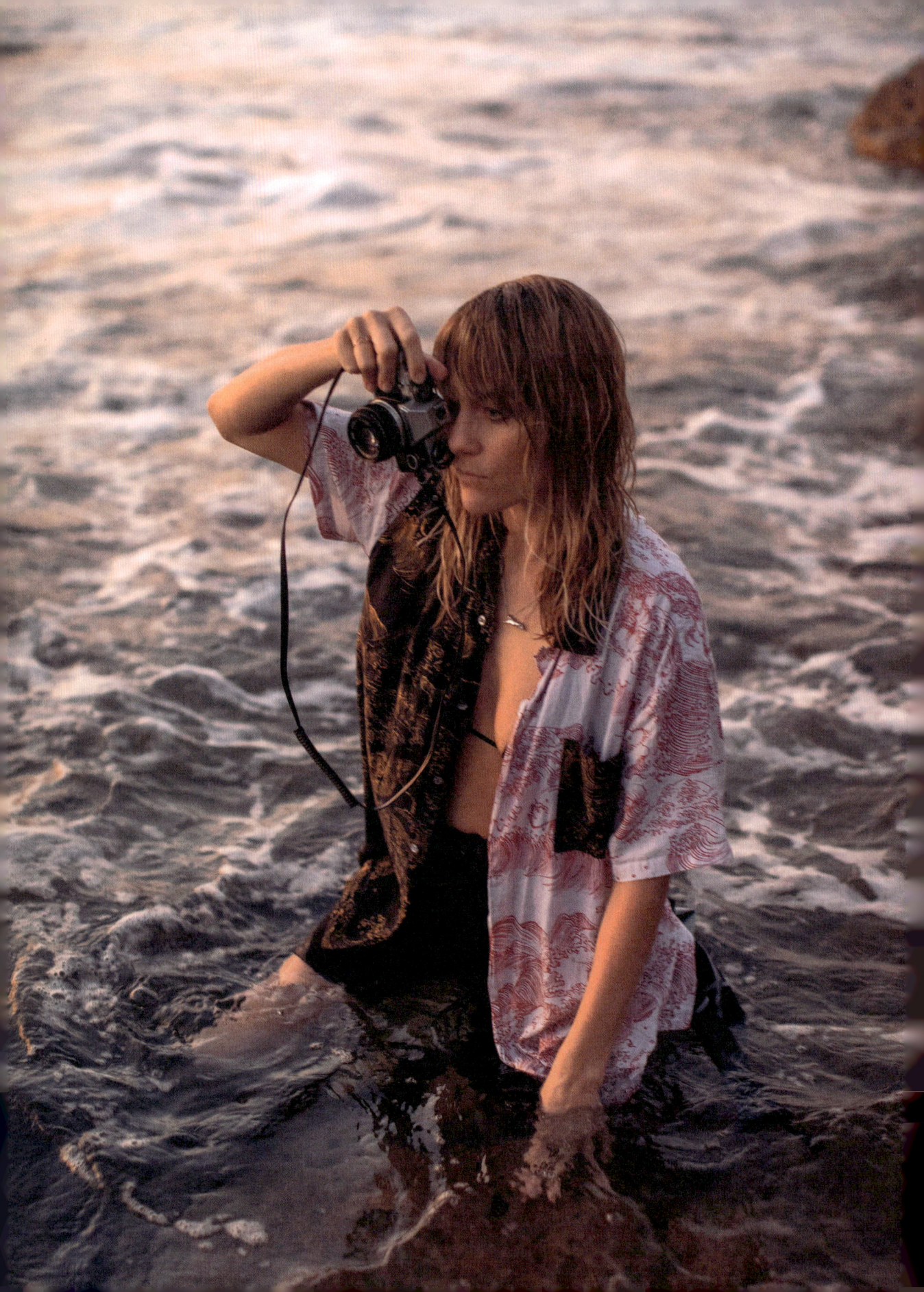

Photography
and filmmaking

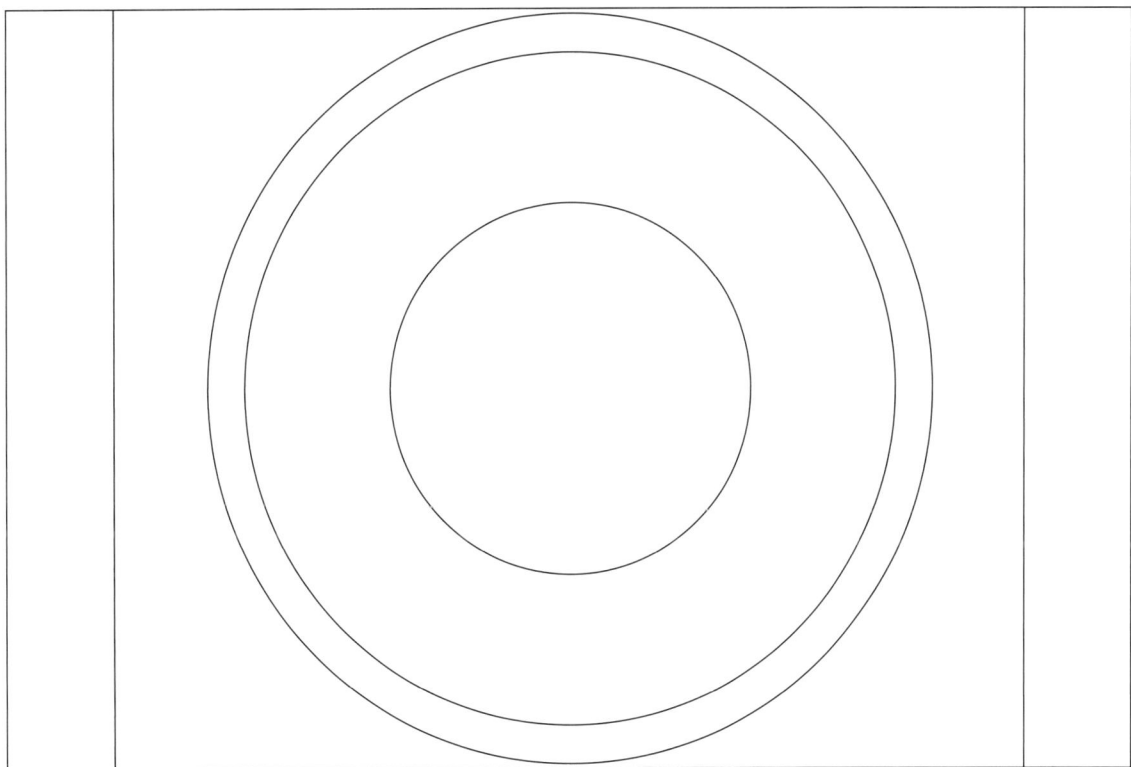

Capturing images to advocate for our oceans and its inhabitants

Alice
Wesley-Smith

● Australia

Capturing beautiful images is a crucial part of Alice Wesley-Smith's work in photography and ocean conservation filmmaking, but with her deep reverence for the ocean, seeing the harsh reality of our reefs and sea animal populations in decline brings a sombre aspect to this work. 'One of the challenges is really understanding what's happening, really keeping your eyes open. That can be extremely confronting,' says Alice.

Originally starting out in the fashion industry, Alice's deep love of the ocean drew her to explore underwater photography. 'Photography on land is hard as it is, then you go underwater, and you've got completely different light conditions; you've got current, swell, a wild environment, and your own physical capabilities,' she says. 'You have to either learn how to hold your breath or master scuba diving equipment and technical skills.' Despite these challenges, seeing her work now, you would assume that Alice had many years of training and guidance rather than being completely self-taught.

Choosing who she works with according to their values and what their business stands for allows Alice to weave her passions for conservation into her creative and professional pursuits. 'I know people don't always have this opportunity but it's really important for me to work with like-minded people; for the people that are doing it for the right reasons, people that are genuinely passionate about conservation and sustainability.' Having her ethics guide her work opportunities has seen Alice join forces with many inspiring organisations.

One example of this style of partnership is with the short film series captured by Alice called *Now You See Me*. In collaboration with Sydney-based jewellery business Sarah & Sebastian, who have pledged to donate one million dollars towards ocean conservation over the next decade, Alice has shot stunningly beautiful footage that dives deep into both Australia's sea lion population and the Great Barrier Reef. These films are available for all to watch online free of charge as a way to encourage more people to care for and connect with the ocean.

Growing up in a creative household, Alice's natural inclination towards photography was obvious and perhaps even expected. But her love of wild natural spaces was something she remembers developing when she was just seven years old on a holiday in Kakadu in Australia's Northern Territory. 'I remember a tropical sky of every colour. The black and purple of an electrical storm coming mixed with a sunset of yellows, pinks and reds. I was blown away and that image stuck with me ever since.'

Now Alice craves getting out into the wildest places she can find. 'I love really sensual, visceral sort of places,' she says. Living in one of the busiest parts of Sydney, Australia, Alice feels the urge to get out of town every couple of weeks. When this isn't possible, she goes searching for natural spaces like walking trails and the beach. 'Getting out in nature doesn't necessarily mean snorkelling or getting in the ocean, just being outside counts. Listen to the crickets at night or the bats flying past. Look at an amazing flower that you hadn't noticed before. Nature is around us all the time.'

Presence is what Alice says is the most important key for connecting with nature. 'When you've got a lens in front of your eye, you're only thinking about capturing it, you're not really looking around and taking in your environment,' she says. 'What you're absorbing is very different. It's important creatively, to put the camera down and be present.' Wise words that many of us can learn to appreciate not only for our creativity but in general life. Most of us could benefit from putting down our technology, experiencing life through our own eyes. 'Small moments are just as impactful as the big moments. Be present with those and appreciate them.'

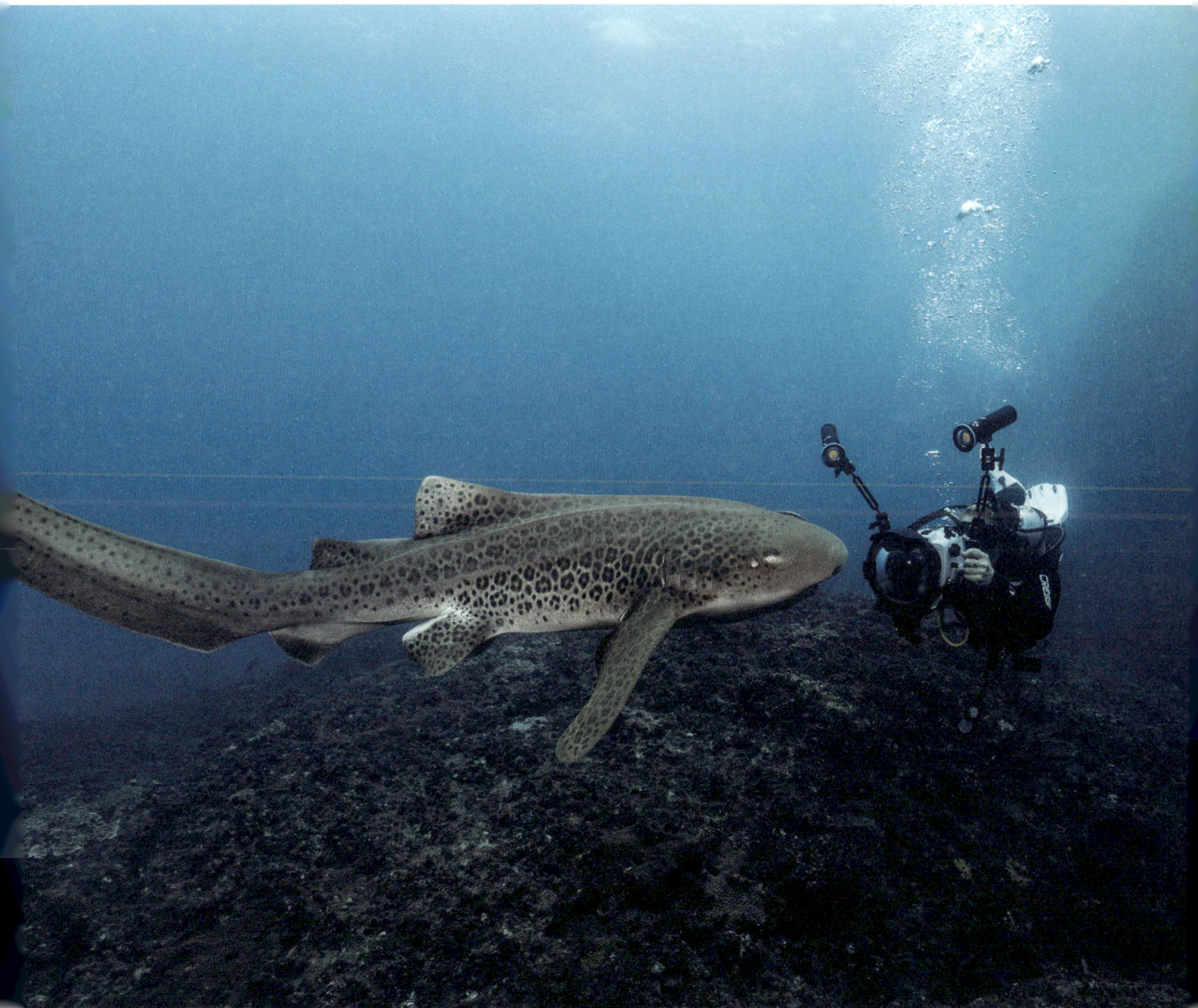

'I think of when I've felt the most connected,
the most free and the most inspired: it's always
in natural spaces.'

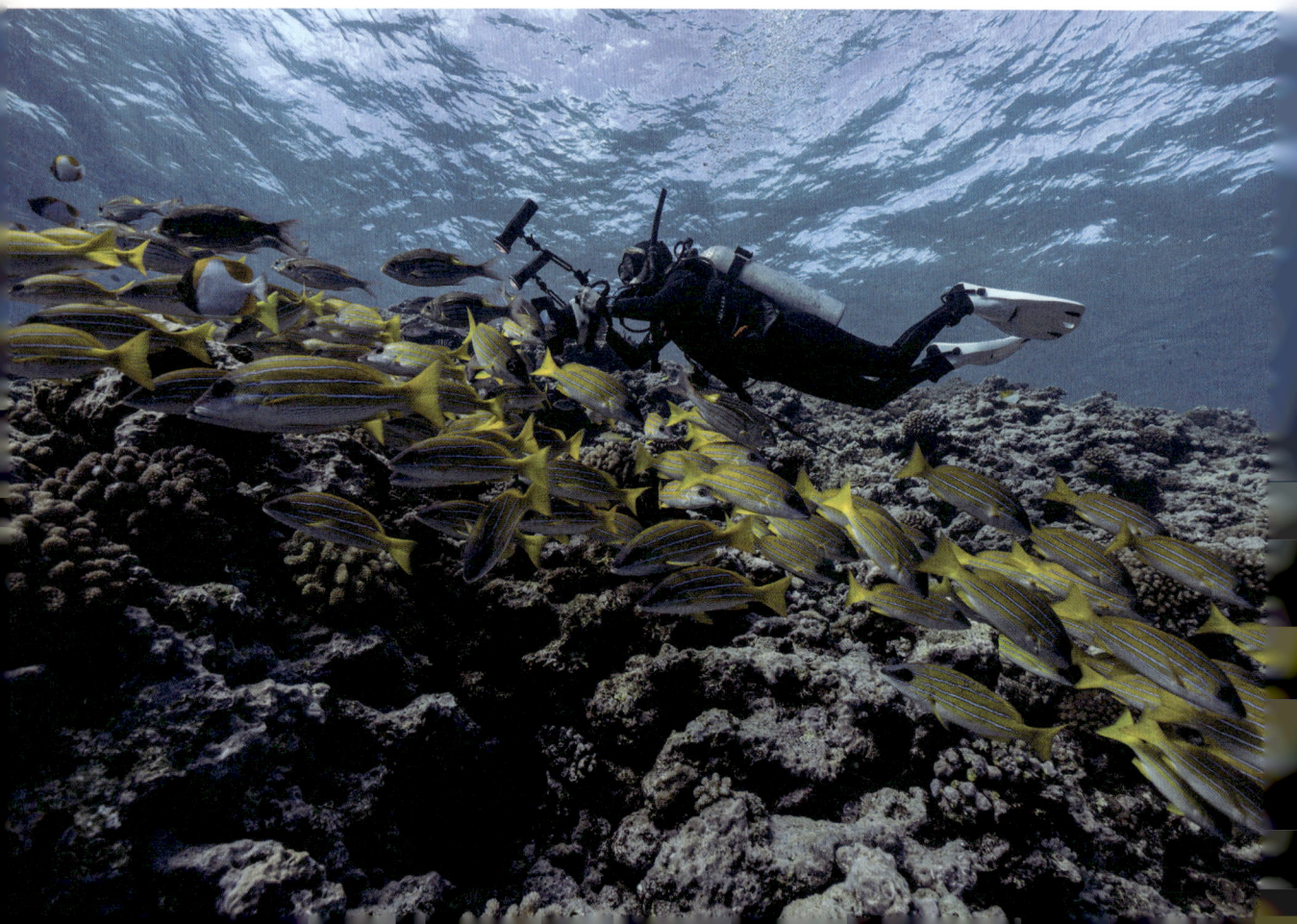

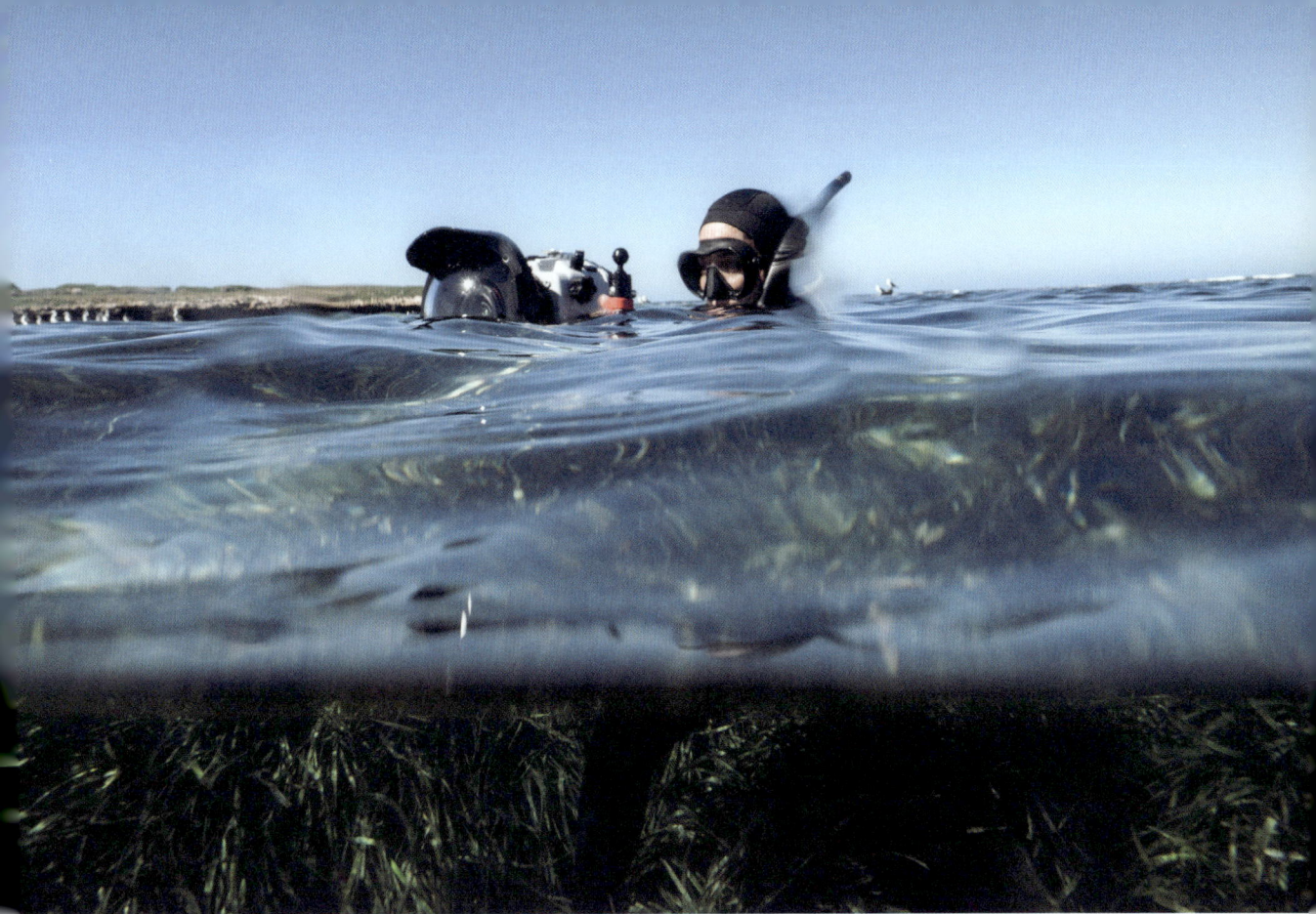

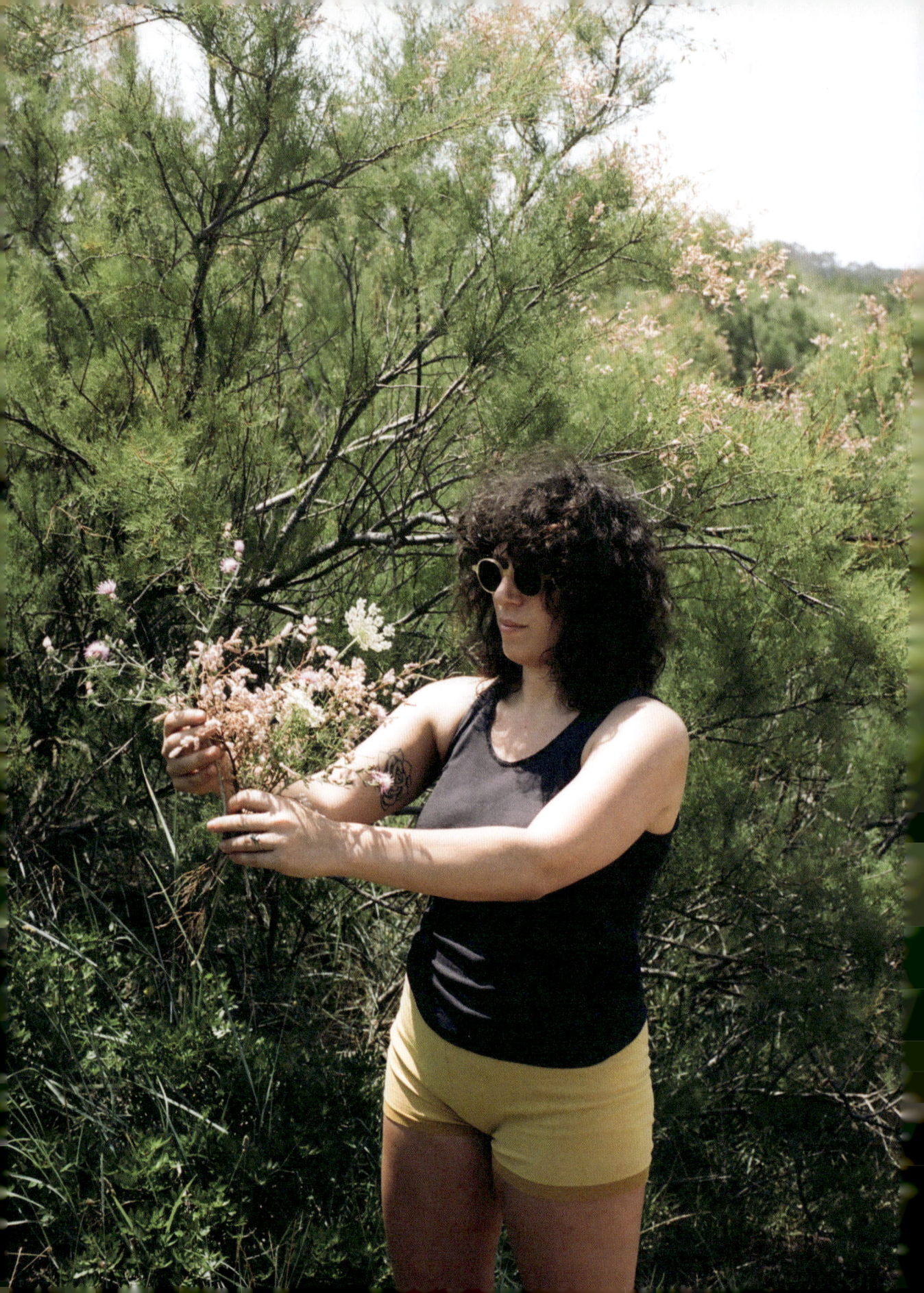

Floristry

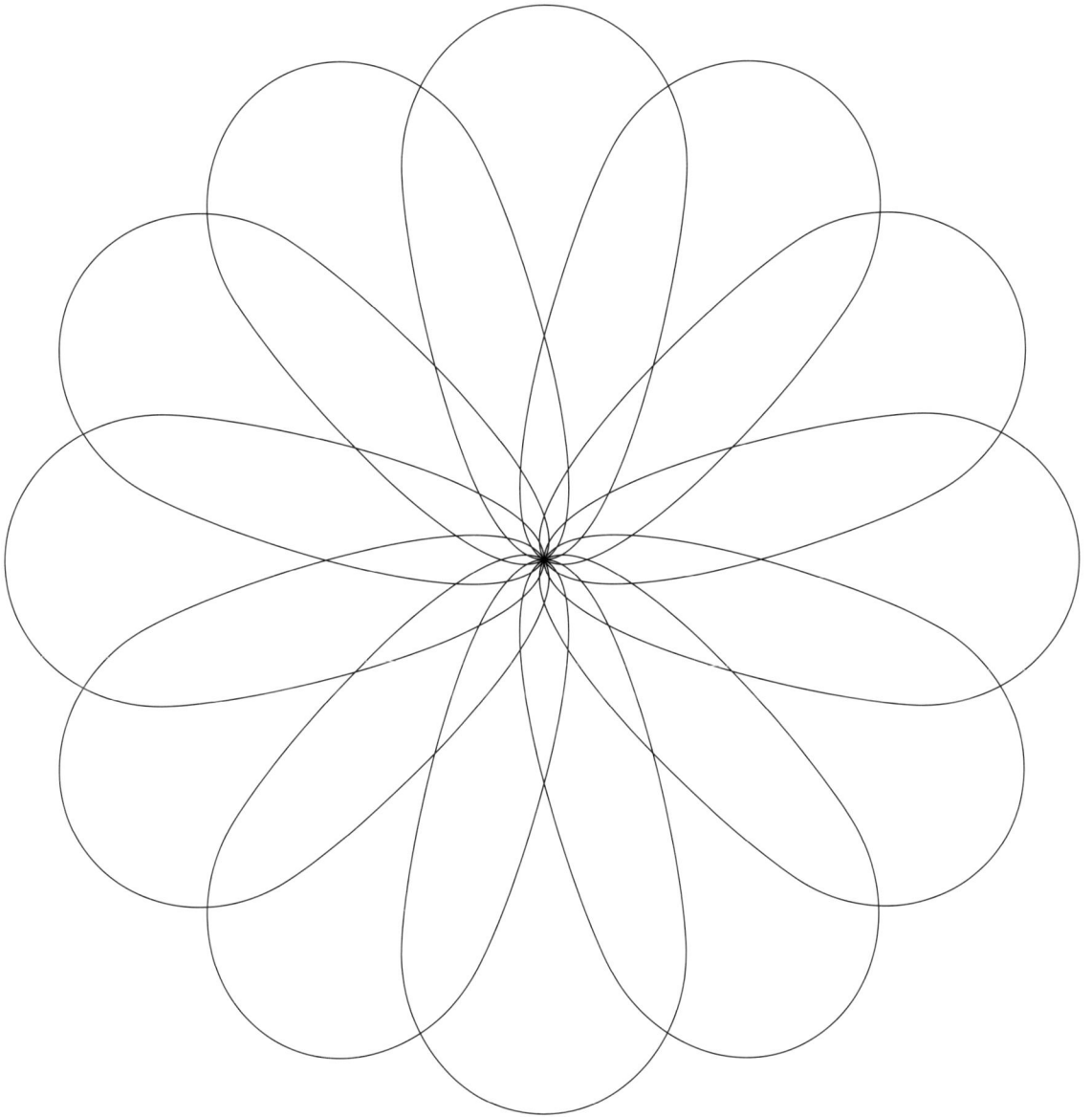

Using flowers to influence emotions

Sophie Wolanski

● Australia

Sophie Wolanski never thought she was a creative person, but using flowers and foliage has helped to strengthen this side of her. She describes herself as a logical and analytical thinker who thrived in subjects like mathematics in school. However, it was her love of working with her hands and the beauty she found in natural elements when they were going through different stages of growth and decay which eventually led her to pursue floristry.

Sophie's early impressions of creativity were that you could become a photographer or a painter – 'something that fits into an artist box' – however, upon enrolling in a fine arts degree at university, a subject in sculpture completely changed her major and the course of her career. 'Sculpture, in hindsight, informs a lot of what I do and in a reverse way, a lot of things that I made had the same sensibility. Nature was always involved and so I don't have anything to show for that four-year degree,' says Sophie, reflecting back on the impermanence of her main subject matter. The sculptures Sophie made were recreations of natural settings using living materials. She would grow things on pieces of wood and document as various things would decay. All of these sculptures have since rotted and deteriorated away, in a similar way that her arrangements do now.

'Flowers are a completely impermanent thing and everyone has their own interpretation of that. To me, the receiving of the flowers is the bigger part. If I put an amazing flower in an arrangement that gives you a specific feeling but is dead in the morning, maybe that was all that flower was supposed to give you.' This sentiment of Sophie's is not always shared with others who wish, or expect, their flowers to last forever. Nonetheless, it is that initial reaction that people have to flowers that is one of the main reasons why she loves her work.

'Flowers are decor but they are the only piece of decor that hold emotion, they make people feel things and can change the atmosphere of what's going on. Flowers have an incredible impact on people.' This simple act of sending flowers can say 'I'm sorry' or 'I love you', it can show someone you care for them, you're thinking about them and you want to celebrate them. It can make someone feel special.

Interestingly, these emotions are not something she often has the privilege to witness. Sophie loves story building for events such as weddings, which can often be over a year in the making. A relationship is built over this time with the couple, yet, once the flowers are installed, Sophie leaves and doesn't get to see her customers experience their flowers.

Unlike many florists, Sophie didn't grow up in a gardening family but she does remember her house in suburban Sydney, Australia, always filled with beautiful flowers. Her mum would regularly go up to the local florist and ensure their house was stocked with flowers and branches. 'Flowers were a huge part of our daily existence. I used to say my dream career, but not the "real one", would be a florist. I thought it was too hard and the early mornings would be impossible.' Over the years, Sophie has come to love her time at the flower markets as a place to reflect on the seasonality of nature, observing what is available at certain times of the year.

The wonder of nature

Having lived around the world, Sophie recognises that there are stark contrasts between locations and what it means to be seasonal. 'New York is such a cultural melting pot and as a result their market flowers are imported from around the world. So even in the middle of a blizzard there are flowers everywhere.' However, while living in New Zealand Sophie found it hard to get hold of the flowers she wanted. Due to tight biosecurity laws, there are a lot less imported flowers so she evolved her style and relied more on found materials. 'I wouldn't use the more typical stuff because I didn't have access to it. It was a lot more of working outside the box because it had to be.' In Auckland, Sophie drove thirty minutes outside of the city to find grasses, fruit trees and wild roses growing on the side of the highway to use in her work. Even though she would get scratches all up her arms from foraging, this was a process she loved as it would give her a truly unique piece to work with and it would often 'make' the event she was styling.

Having a conscious attitude to the natural world has been the backbone of how Sophie runs her business. Reusing the plastic sleeves and rubber bands her flowers come in and using butcher's paper with twine to wrap her bouquets are just second nature now. On reflecting about her decision to not have a shopfront or hold stock, Sophie says, 'At the beginning it was detrimental to my profit but things are definitely turning around now.' Choosing to create-to-order and working mainly on larger-scale events means less flowers are going in the bin.

For budding florists, Sophie suggests trying to find sustainable ways of doing things as a show of respect for the flowers and for the planet. 'It's important to know that flowers are a living and dying thing and that they won't last forever. We are taking these things that have been in nature and rearranging them into something else for the rest of their lives.'

'If I put an amazing flower in an arrangement that gives you a specific feeling but is dead in the morning, maybe that was all that flower was supposed to give you.'

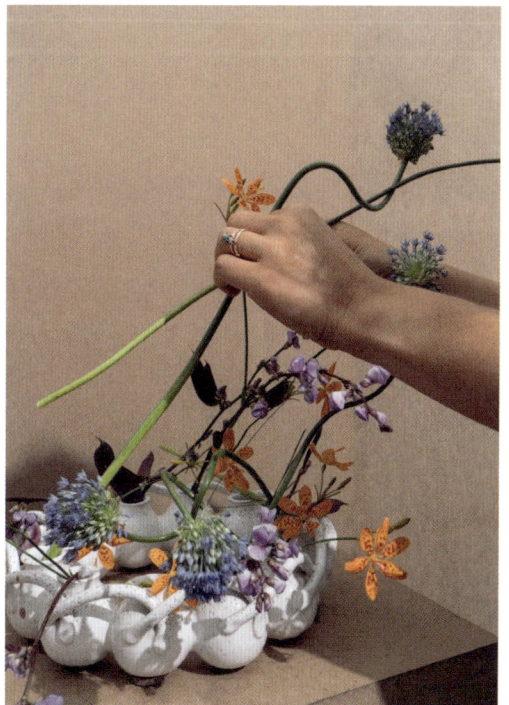

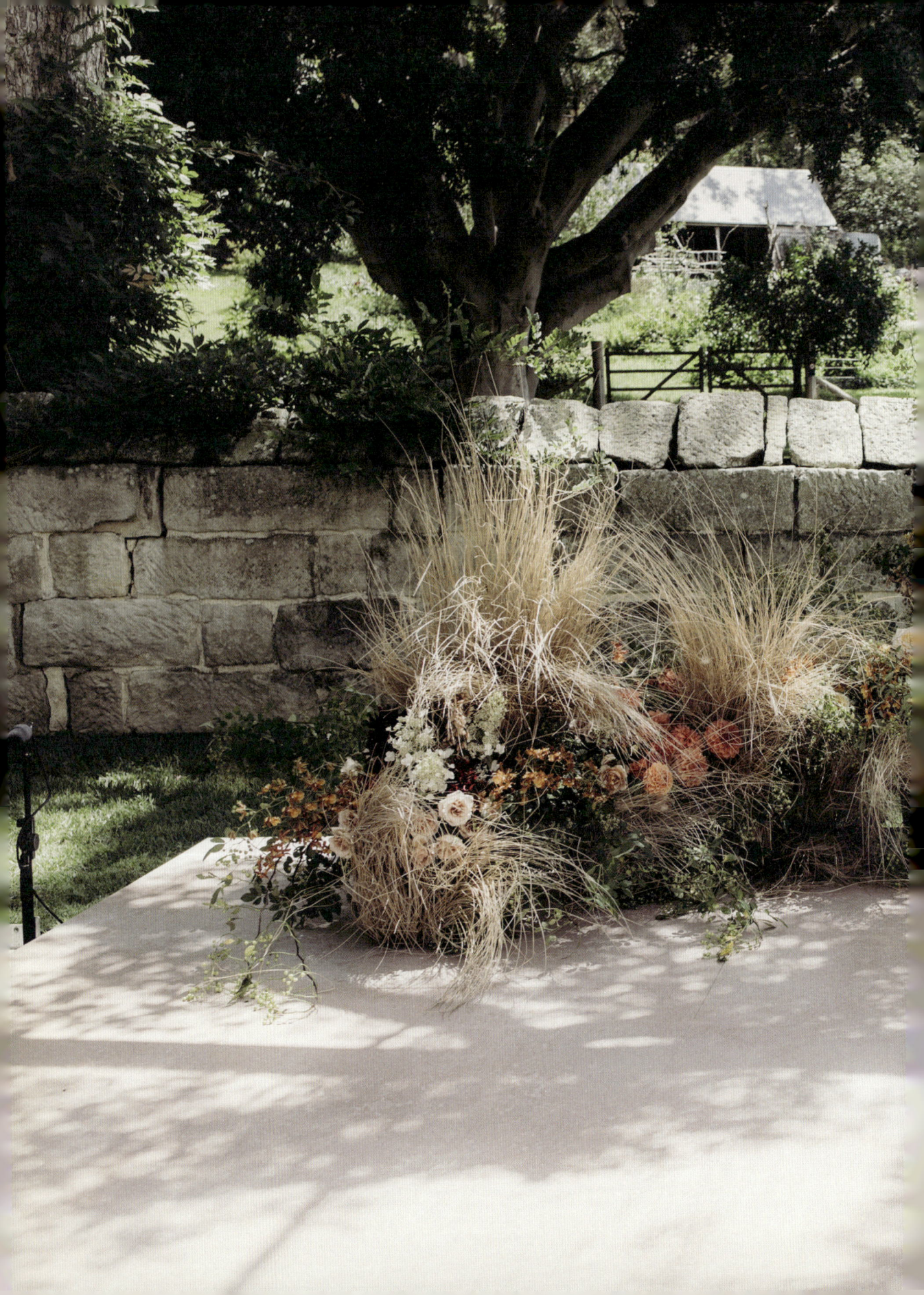

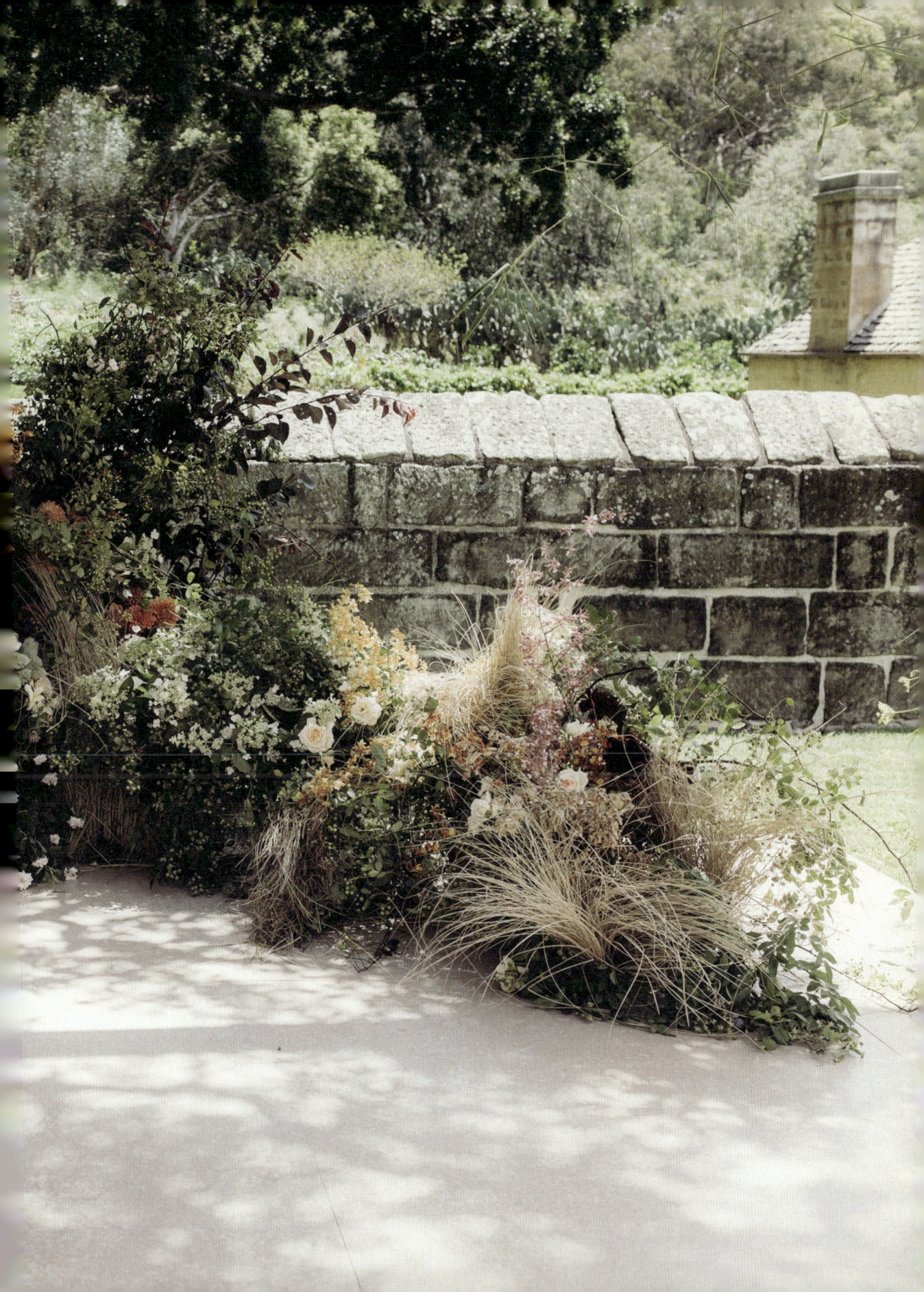

Findings

When I embarked on this journey, I couldn't wait to speak with all of these different women and to hear their histories, their adventures and all of the things they have learnt on their journeys. Some of these women I've known of and dreamed of meeting for a very long time. Others I found along the way thanks to the mention of a name from a friend, the collaboration with someone I admire or simply by chance, coming across their work as though I had accidentally stumbled upon a pot of gold at the end of a rainbow.

What I didn't expect from this process was to hear similar threads of wisdom woven through each woman's story. How could such a diverse group of women from every continent on this Earth all have such parallel lessons to share? When I would ask these women questions, I was excited by the potential of hearing something new. But halfway through I began to realise that there is more potency in the similarities of these women rather than the differences. A kinship of women.

And so, while I suggest reading every story individually and connecting to the women who you feel spark your inner light, I'd like to share the major lessons of this collection of stories with you in the hope that, if nothing else, you can see some relevance for nurturing these in your own life.

● Community

Being part of a community of people is essential for our survival. Humans are not meant to be solitary beings, we thrive off connection with others – both from a survival standpoint and for our enjoyment.

I can't imagine not having the women I work with to bounce ideas off, share interesting research we've found or discuss tricky cases with. Finding your community, a group of like-minded people, is essential for thriving.

Many of the women in this book were pioneers, creating their own communities and paving the way for others to feel safe to explore activities never before available to them. By following their dreams, they showed others how they too could follow theirs.

Community also extends to being part of the natural world. We are not separate from nature, we are just as much a part of nature as the trees, the rivers and the sky. We belong to the community of nature.

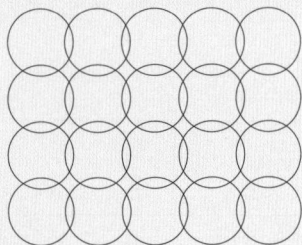

● Curiosity

Having an open and curious mind is the foundation for learning something new. When I asked each of these women what advice they would give to the reader for building a strong connection to nature, more than half replied 'just try it'.

No one is born a painter, or a surfer, or a chef. These skills are fostered from curiosity. Something intrigues us so we try it out, we decide that we like it and off we go. Unless we try something for the first time, we will never know how it makes us feel.

My curiosity to heal my own body naturally from pain and hormonal challenges is what helped me to become the naturopath that I am today. Without wanting to explore something new, I would likely not be writing this book.

You don't need to have a family history or working background in any area to want to try it out. You can be curious about anything, but being curious about nature means that you are curious about life.

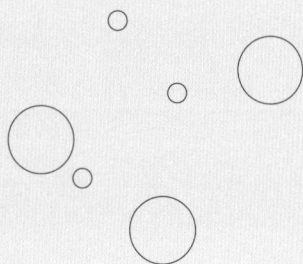

● Healing

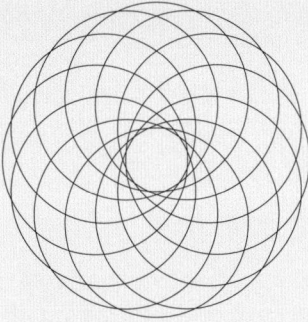

Being part of the natural world is inherently healing. Whether you are recovering from an injury, experiencing grief or are suffering from the stresses of modern life. Nature can be a soothing balm to many ailments.

Spending time alone with the natural world has been part of Indigenous cultures around the world for thousands of years for good reason. Before many of our modern diseases took over, most of what we needed for good health could be found in the elements.

But we do not need to be sick to experience healing. Wellness is infinite. I love when women come to me wanting to improve their health. They are not all in a crisis or suffering. Many simply want to explore their body's potential.

Growth is available to all of us. You don't see a healthy plant just stop growing; it may not get taller but it will continue expanding, blooming and evolving. We have that same opportunity.

● Patience

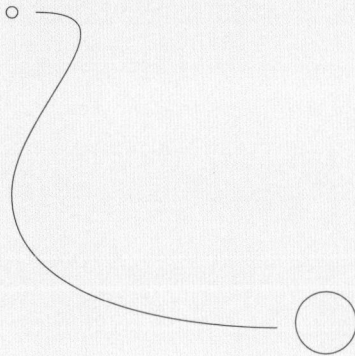

You cannot rush a vegetable to grow, a wave to come or rain to fall. We must wait patiently. In a world that is set up for efficiency and convenience, taking our time is a skill many of us have lost.

In my work, I always preface that the process is gradual and nonlinear. There is no diet or herb that will give you overnight results. You must surrender to the journey, commit to the path and allow the body time to rebalance.

What can slowing down teach us? Or rather, what do we miss when we don't slow down? If we are constantly in a hurry multitasking and enhancing processes so that we no longer have to wait for anything, we miss out on the joy of simply being.

If we are rushing through life, we are going to miss it. When we spend time around animals, in the forest or by the water, we soon realise how uncomfortable we feel when we slow down. Challenging that discomfort takes patience.

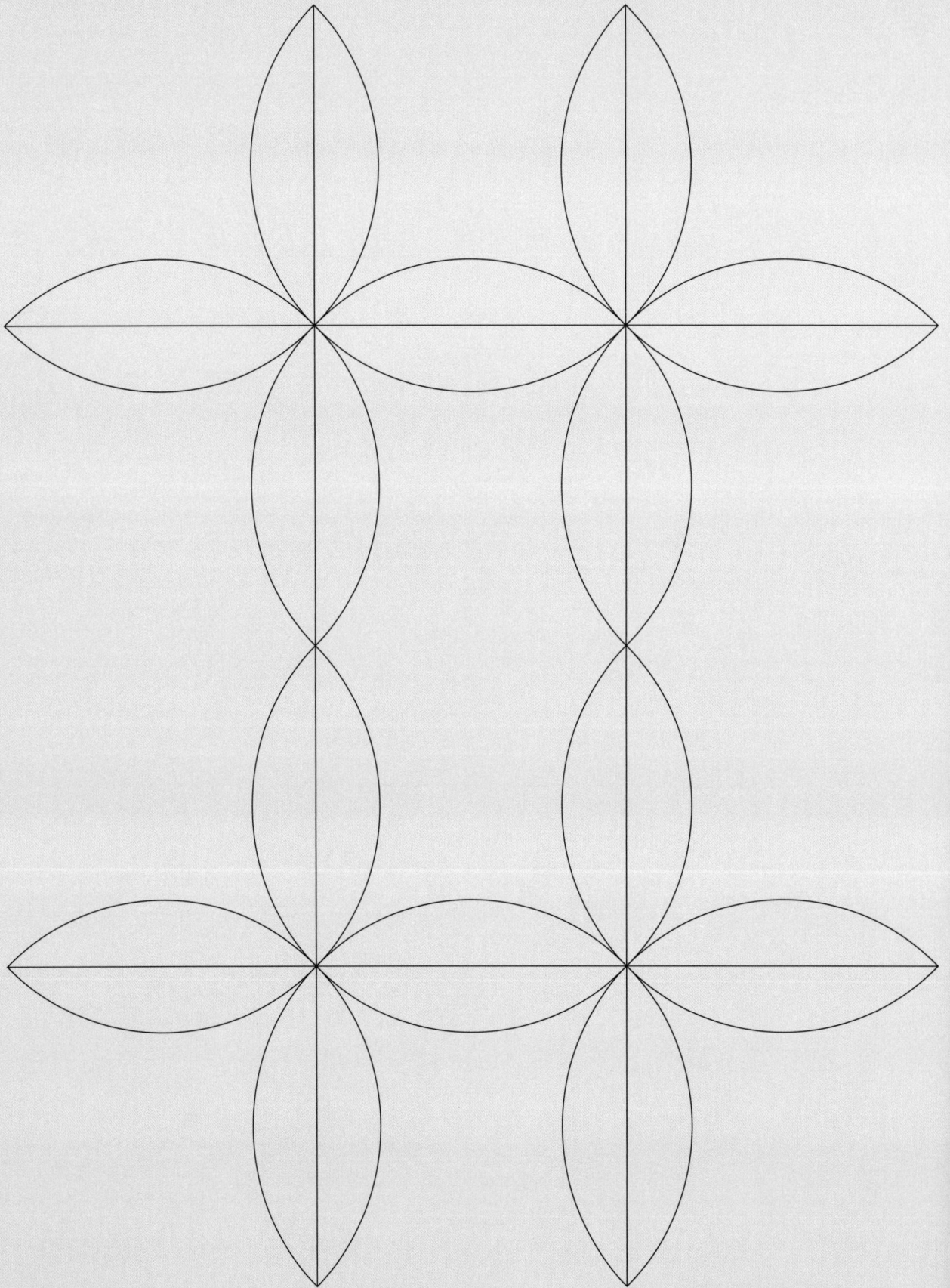

Nature first-aid kit

If your lifestyle is really busy and you are struggling to fit in new activities:

Pick one of the 'for the now' activities to do each day (these only take a couple of minutes) and one of the 'for the future' activities to do each month.

If you have a little more time up your sleeve:

Try to incorporate two or more of the 'for the now' activities into your daily schedule and one of the 'for the future' activities every week.

$\longrightarrow$

● For the now

If you have a headache, you're feeling tired, unmotivated, cranky or stressed, this section is for you. When you need a 'quick fix' to get you out of your funk, pick one of these simple but powerful remedies. Each one should take no longer than a few minutes of your time, meaning you can do one on your lunch break, during your child's naptime or between tasks. See the Plant meditation on page 70 for additional inspiration.

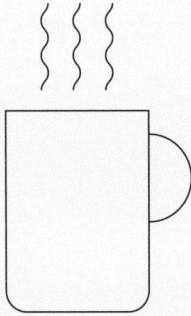

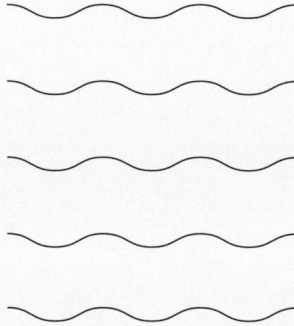

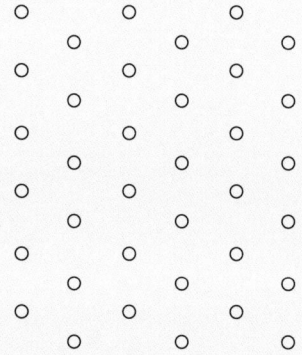

● Herbal tea

Brew yourself a cup of herbal tea. If you have fresh peppermint or lemon balm, pick 3–4 leaves per cup. For ginger tea, I suggest half a knob of thinly sliced ginger with a squeeze of lemon and a drizzle of honey. Otherwise, opt for a teaspoon of your favourite dried herb (mine is chamomile). Don't do anything else while you drink your tea, sip mindfully and slowly.

● Fresh air

It sounds simple but get outside. It doesn't matter where you go but remove yourself from indoor spaces for a few minutes. If possible, get a bit of sun on your skin, drink in some fresh air and look around for something natural. If it's raining, maybe allow some water to touch your hand or face. A few moments out of stuffy air and artificial light can be deeply invigorating.

● Grounding

The practice of taking your shoes off and standing on the ground barefoot is referred to as grounding. This should be done on natural surfaces such as sand, grass, dirt or smooth rock. Stand still and feel the whole surface of your feet touching the ground. Maybe it feels warm, maybe there is something between your toes, maybe it tickles. Allow yourself to feel completely supported by Earth. Try doing this between meetings or on your lunch break.

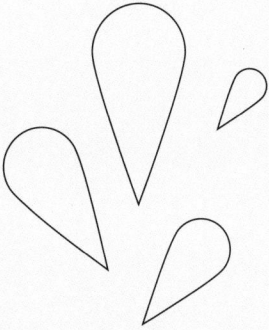

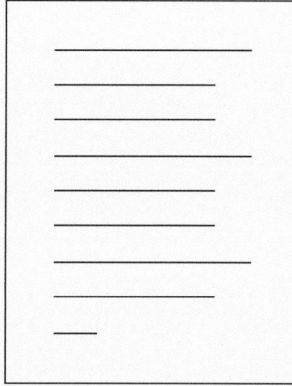

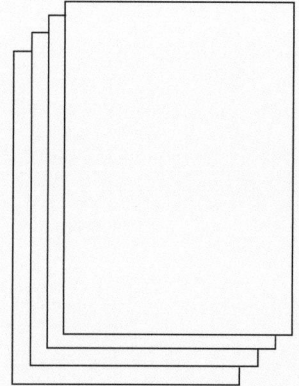

Splash of water

Using cold water from a tap, water bottle – or if you are close to the ocean, a river or lake – splash your face with two handfuls of water. Let the water drip down your face and wake you up. This is great if you are feeling tired or struggling to concentrate. If you are lucky enough to have access to a swimmable patch of water, submerge your body. In the words of Alice Wesley-Smith, 'you'll never regret a swim'.

Nature-based poem

Reading a poem about nature is a powerful way of transporting you into a new environment. I suggest keeping your favourites saved somewhere on your phone or a book in your handbag to refer to when you need it. My favourites are *When I am Among the Trees* by Mary Oliver and *The Road Not Taken* by Robert Frost.

Image library

Viewing images of nature can bring about a sense of calm. Keep a folder in your phone or on your desktop of your favourite nature images. Landscapes, animals or perhaps places you have been. Take a few moments to close all of your other tabs and immerse yourself in these images.

● For the future

In naturopathy we often say that prevention is better than cure. To avoid getting to a state of health that requires treatment we must incorporate certain tools and techniques into our lifestyle. These nature remedies below are accessible for most of us, with some requiring a little more effort than others. If we go to the gym once, we won't see our muscles grow, but if we go regularly over a few months we start to see our body change. These activities work like that, they are the things that continue compounding in their benefits over time.

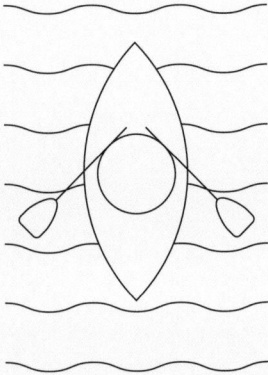

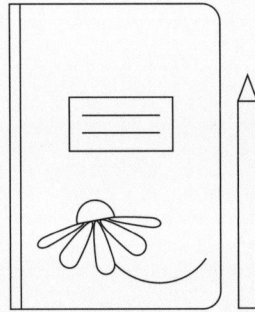

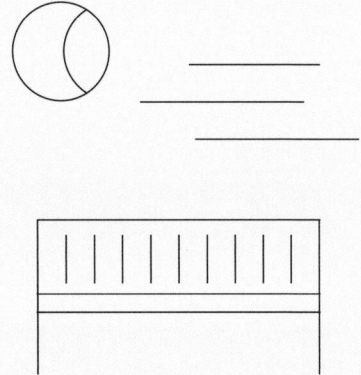

● Outdoor exercise

While many classes and weight-based routines are not often available for us to do outdoors, there are many other forms of exercise we can incorporate into our lifestyle. Walking, running, cycling, rowing, kayaking, surfing, paddleboarding and a huge portion of team sports are offered outdoors. Try swapping one of your indoor exercises for something outside each week.

● Nature drawing

Landscapes, animals and plants can be deeply inspiring for creativity. If you don't think you are a creative person or this is an area you want to strengthen, I recommend taking a notebook and a pencil for a walk somewhere in nature. Find something that catches your eye – a flower, leaf or view – and with no rush, start drawing. It doesn't have to be perfect as it is simply your interpretation of what you are seeing. More details are on page 126.

● Sit spot

As explained on page 39, the sit spot is a place out in nature that you return to regularly over time. The purpose is to observe and become more familiar with the area, to almost become part of the local environment. It allows an expansion of your awareness, a softness when interacting with the natural world and a deepening of respect for nature.

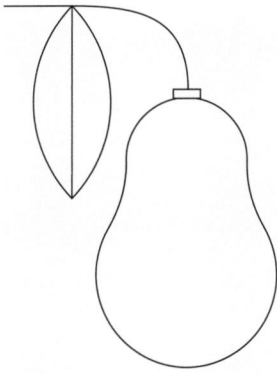

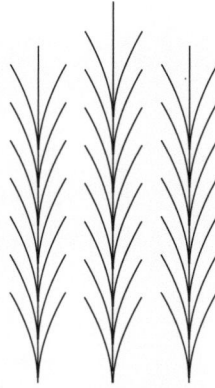

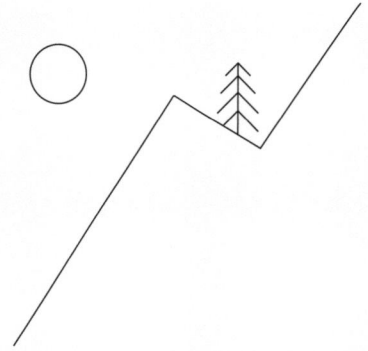

Gardening

There are few things more rewarding than watching a seed you plant in soil turn into a vegetable that you can eventually consume. If you don't have a backyard, you can use a small pot on a windowsill or balcony to grow herbs and flowers. If that still isn't an option try an indoor plant. Caring for and watching your plant grow can be hugely therapeutic for slowing down and paying attention, as well as nourishing for your body.

Foraging

Depending on where you live, you might be able to find a plethora of edible foods just outside your doorstep. Where I live there are mulberry trees, rosemary shrubs and nasturtium bushes all around my suburb as well as community gardens full of fresh fruits, vegetables and herbs. Find a local edible plant resource online or at a library to learn about what plants are in your area. Remember to never take the first or last of anything and double check the safety of anything before you consume it. If you are unsure, leave it untouched.

Hiking

The benefits of hiking are far more than improving our fitness. Spending time immersed in a natural environment is what the Japanese have termed *shinrin-yoku*, also known as forest bathing. By choosing a bush track, a trail along the coast or a loop of your closest parkland, you are allowing yourself to be completely surrounded by nature. Just like Tiina Nopanen tells us on page 44, it doesn't have to be a long trek. A short stroll can be just as beneficial.

→

For the future (continued)

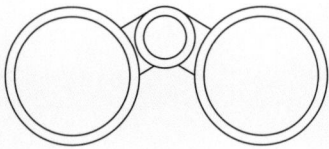

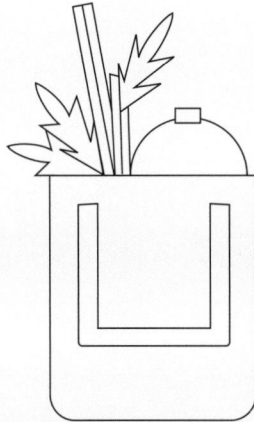

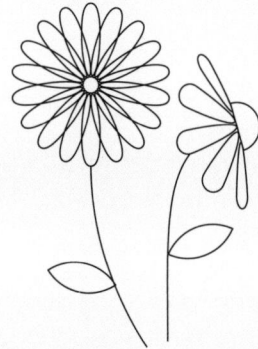

Nature-based trips

If you are lucky enough to get some time off, try taking a trip that revolves around nature. Perhaps it is driving up or down the coast with the windows down and salty air cooling your skin. Take a tent to your closest national park or state forest that allows camping and stay the night to look up at the stars. Climb that mountain you've had on your bucket list, visit the lake you've seen photos of and take your binoculars to spot the rare bird you've read about.

Farmers' market

Most metropolitan areas have a farmers' market. By visiting each week for your produce, you can start to build a relationship with the sellers and learn about their growing practices. This is also a wonderful way of appreciating the seasons. You will likely notice the influx of blueberries in spring, only to disappear and be replaced by tomatoes in summer, apples in autumn, and so on. Read Ria Ibrahim Taylor's story on page 30 for more information on the benefits of understanding the seasons.

Flower arranging

You don't need to spend big money on fancy bouquets to get joy from flowers. If you have a garden (or a friendly neighbour gives you the okay), clip a couple of your favourite blooms and put them into a vase, jar or bottle. I don't recommend cutting from private land or council areas but anything that has fallen on the ground is fair game. Like Sophie Wolanski on page 158, you can think outside of the box for your bunch and get experimental with shapes and textures. A hand-picked bouquet, in my opinion, is also far more sentimental as a gift than something pre-prepared from a store.

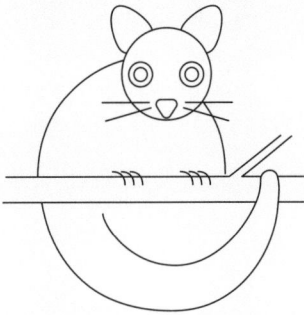

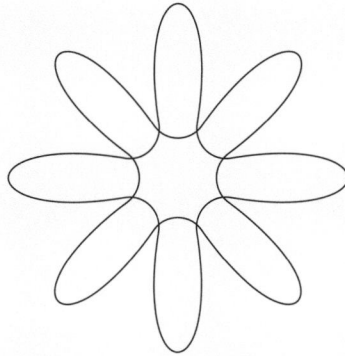

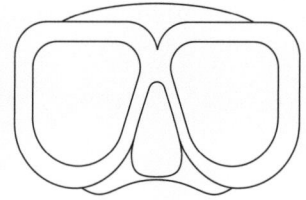

Animal connection

This is easy if you have a pet but if not, go outside and find an animal. As mentioned in more detail on page 137, it does not matter what type of animal you pick – it can be as little as a beetle or a sparrow. Watch what this animal is doing, follow its movements and see how it interacts with its environment or fellow animals. If you return to the same spot repeatedly, you might see the same animal again. Just like a neighbour, you begin to form a relationship with this animal and an appreciation for its place in your world.

Naturopathy

The practice of naturopathy is about helping others reach their optimal health with the use of natural therapies. This might be herbal medicine, nutritional advice or lifestyle support. For chronic health conditions, especially pertaining to women's bodies, naturopathy can be a wonderfully gentle yet effective way to work towards health. I suggest finding a qualified practitioner to support you through this process. In Australia naturopaths should have a four-year Bachelor of Health Science degree, but qualifications vary internationally.

Try something new

For many of the women in this book, there was a little spark of curiosity that led them to their greatest passion. Have you always wanted to try scuba diving? Book a class! Have you been intrigued by rock climbing? Sign up for a lesson! If it's a little out of your reach, perhaps watch a documentary or follow some people on social media who are doing it. Learn what you can and when you are able to, try it for yourself. Humans have come up with so many wonderful ways of interacting with the natural world, wouldn't it be a shame to not give it a go for yourself?

Index of contributors

● website
▲ instagram

Gab Abell 110
● studiumessentials.com
▲ studium.essentials

Wai'ala Ahn 116
▲ petalsandpigments

Kobi Bloom 52
▲ wilderway

Ariella Daly 72
● honeybeewild.com
▲ beekeepinginskirts

Claire Dunn 34
● naturesapprentice.com.au

Giuliana Furci 128
● ffungi.org
▲ giulifungi
▲ fungifoundation

Analiese Gregory 24
● analiesegregory.com
▲ analiesegregory

Rosemary Gladstar 64
● scienceandartofherbalism.com
▲ rosemarygladstar

Melissa Groo 132
● melissagroo.com
▲ melissagroo

Autumn Kitchens 46
▲ autumnkitchens

Jacqui Lanarus & Gab Banay 96
● yolkydokey.com.au
▲ yolkydokey

Glenda McCulloch 146
● cungelellaart.com
▲ cungelellaart
▲ _myrrdah_

Rhiannon Mitchell 106
● saltwatersistas.com.au
▲ saltwater__sistas

Anya Lily Montague 84
● meadowsweet-retreat.com
▲ meadowsweetretreat
▲ anyalily

Zandi Ndhlovu 140
● blackmermaid.co.za
▲ zandithemermaid
▲ theblackmermaid_foundation

Tiina Nopanen 42
▲ toinenjalkaulkona

Paige Northwood 120
● paigenorthwood.com
▲ paigenorthwood

Samorn Sanixay 102
▲ samorn_sanixay

Leah Scott 12
● leahscott.net
▲ leahscottie

Aysha Sharif 78
● thewanderlustwomen.co.uk
▲ the.wanderlust.women
▲ amira_thewanderlust

Mitzi Jonelle Tan 58
▲ mitzijonelle

Ria Ibrahim Taylor 30
● soulfirefarm.org
▲ soulfirefarm

Alice Wesley-Smith 150
● alicewesleysmith.com
▲ alicewesleysmith

Sophie Wolanski 156
● muckfloral.com
▲ muckfloral

To the women

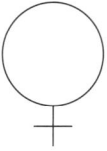

I want to acknowledge all the women who aren't featured in this book. The women who didn't have time to be interviewed, who didn't respond to or see my requests for interviews, who I never came across in my research. You are all important and if I could have met every single woman doing something amazing in, with and for nature, this would be a mighty thick book.

I wholeheartedly tried to include as diverse a group as I could find and to keep the term 'woman' open to those who were both assigned female at birth and those who identify as women. I chose to focus on women because that's who I work with and that's who I am, it is my closest community and audience. I do not disregard the experiences of other genders and their relationship with nature, that just wasn't my book.

I also want to acknowledge the importance of the many women on this Earth, particularly of Indigenous cultures, who have deep relationships with nature. To those women, the trailblazers, I thank you. You are our example.

To the twenty-five intelligent, creative, beautiful, fierce and inspiring women who I did get to meet, I give my deepest gratitude. I am intrinsically changed from this experience. The stories and images expressed in these pages can hardly translate the wisdom and reverence these women share with the world. It is my sincerest hope that they all continue to bloom in their respective roles as guardians of the natural world, spreading their seeds of truth and helping others feel grounded in their place.

Acknowledgements

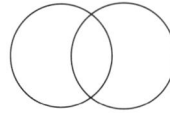

Thank you to all the women in my life who have supported me. To my mum who is always encouraging and proud even when she doesn't really know what it is that I'm writing. To my beautiful friends Sarah, Tash, Lara, Lucy, Liz, Haylee, Steph and Mim, who showed me so much enthusiasm and shared my excitement every step of the way.

To Nina for your guidance and mentorship, without you, this book would quite literally never have happened. To Kirsten Abbott, Shannon Grey, Lisa Schuurman, and the team of women at Thames & Hudson who brought this book to life and made it beautiful. To all of the women I've ever worked with, will work with or may never get the chance to work with, thank you. This is for you.

Special thank you to my partner, Cam, who witnessed the highs and lows of writing this book, wrestling with my own lifestyle and choices. Without you as a pillar to lean on I may have fallen apart or never finished. You allowed me to lean into the value of this message and my worthiness to share it.

And to you, the reader, thank you for taking the time to immerse yourself in the wonders of nature. The animals, the water, the plants, Earth and most of all, the people who make up nature are here for you. If you now gaze at a flower a little longer or wiggle your toes in the dirt a little more often, my job here is done.

First published in Australia in 2023
by Thames & Hudson Australia Pty Ltd
11 Central Boulevard, Portside Business Park
Port Melbourne, Victoria 3207
ABN: 72 004 751 964

First published in the United Kingdom in 2024
by Thames & Hudson Ltd
181a High Holborn
London WC1V 7QX

First published in the United States of America in 2024
by Thames & Hudson Inc.
500 Fifth Avenue
New York, New York 10110

Women & Nature © Thames & Hudson Australia 2023
Women Who Heal © Thames & Hudson Australia 2023

Text © Emma Drady
Images © copyright remains with the individual
copyright holders

Image credits
Title page: Jacki Bruniquel (p. 2); Introduction:
Abby Ferguson (p. 6); The practice of nature:
Josh Burkinshaw (p. 12), Nana Cascardo (p. 15),
Majell Backhausen (p. 16), Jodie McBride (pp. 17–9); Tom
Roberts (pp. 24, 27), Jonah Vitale-Wolff (pp. 28, 33),
Gabriela Álvarez (p. 32), Ben Ey for Australian Geographic
(pp. 34, 37), Tiina Nopanen (pp. 42, 45), Autumn Winters
(p. 46), Greg Fulks (pp. 49, 51), Life of Riley NYC (p. 50),
Robbie Warden (pp. 52, 57), Tim Carroll (p. 55), Esther
Paige (p. 56), Youth Advocates for Climate Action
Phillipines (pp. 58, 61); The wisdom of nature: Danielle
Cohen (pp. 64, 67), Onyx Baird (pp. 72, 75), Koa Kalish
(p. 76), Amira Patel (pp. 78, 81–2), Adam Raja (p. 83),
Cecilia Renard (pp. 84, 88–91), Jacqui Lanarus & Gab
Banay (pp. 96–101), Tom Greenwood Photography (p. 102),
Samorn Sanixay (p. 105, bottom), Dr David Wong
(p. 105, top), Wayila Creative (pp. 106, 109), Andrea Lane
(p. 110), Oliver Kleyn (p. 113, right), Gab Abell (p. 113, left);
The wonder of nature: Abby Ferguson (pp. 116, 119),
Paige Northwood (pp. 120, 123), Mateo Barrenengoa
(pp. 128, 131), Michael Forsberg Photography (p. 132),
Melissa Groo (p. 135), Nicolene Olckers (p. 140), Jacki
Bruniquel (pp. 143–45), Sarah Conlan Photography (p. 146),
Cheryl Perez (p. 149), Kasia Werstak (p. 150), Sarah Munro
(pp. 153–55), Rob Champion (p. 156), This Humid House
(p. 159), Sophie Wolanski (pp. 160–61).

26 25 24 23   5 4 3 2 1

Thames & Hudson Australia wishes to acknowledge that
Aboriginal and Torres Strait Islander people are the first
storytellers of this nation and the Traditional Custodians of
the land on which we live and work. We acknowledge their
continuing culture and pay respect to Elders past, present
and future.

ISBN 978-1-760-76368-8 (hardback)
ISBN 978-1-760-76404-3 (U.S. edition)

A catalogue record for this
book is available from the
National Library of Australia

British Library Cataloguing-in-Publication Data
A catalogue record for this book is available from the
British Library

Library of Congress Control Number 2023938537

Every effort has been made to trace accurate ownership
of copyrighted text and visual materials used in this book.
Errors or omissions will be corrected in subsequent
editions, provided notification is sent to the publisher.

Front cover: Ashlea O'Neill | Salt Camp Studio
Photo: Cecilia Renard

Design: Ashlea O'Neill | Salt Camp Studio
Editing: Lisa Schuurman
Printed and bound in China by C&C Offset
Printing Co., Ltd

FSC® is dedicated to the promotion of responsible forest
management worldwide. This book is made of material
from FSC®-certified forests and other controlled sources.

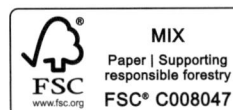

MIX
Paper | Supporting
responsible forestry
FSC® C008047

Be the first to know about our new releases,
exclusive content and author events by visiting
thamesandhudson.com.au
thamesandhudson.com
thamesandhudsonusa.com

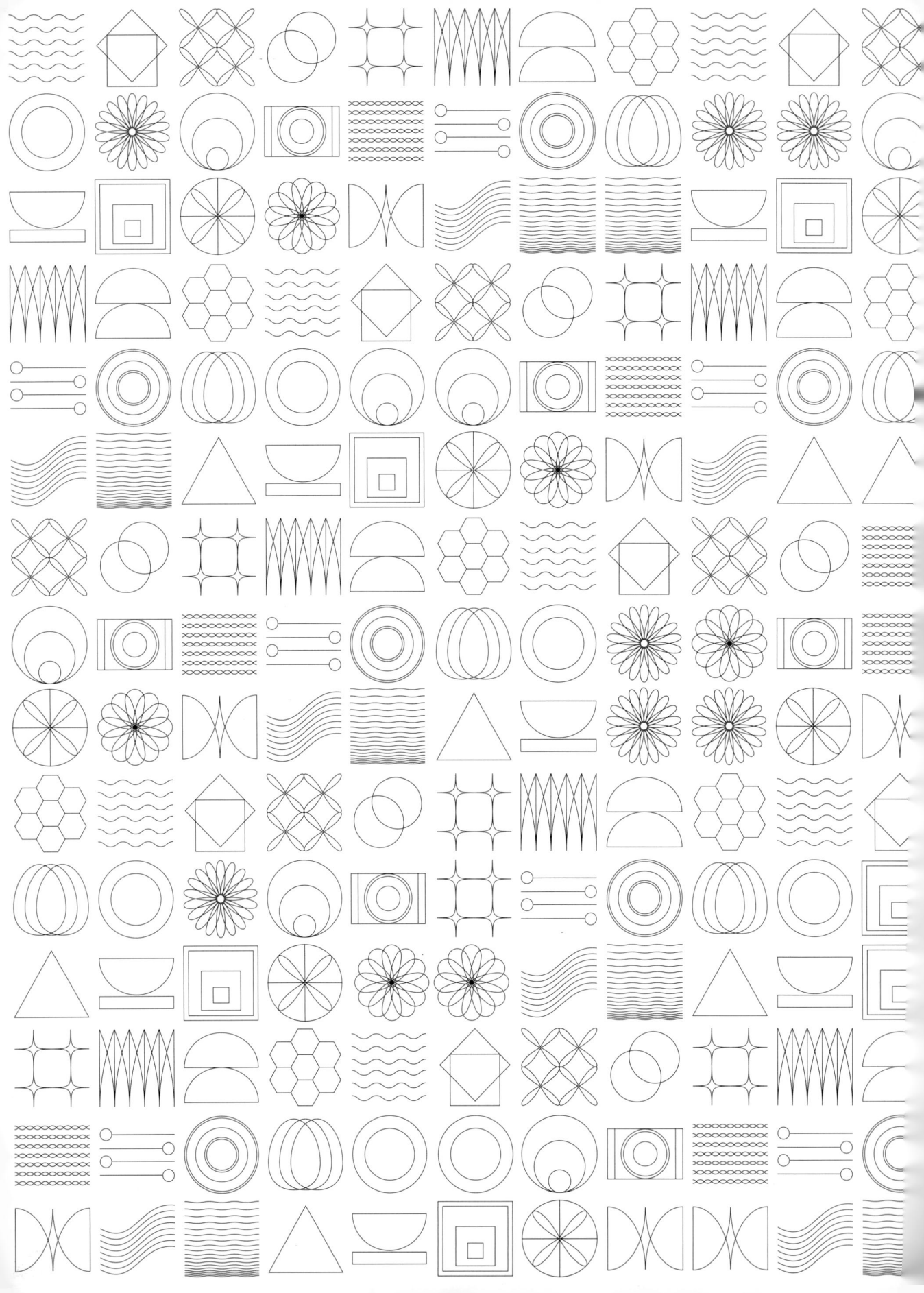